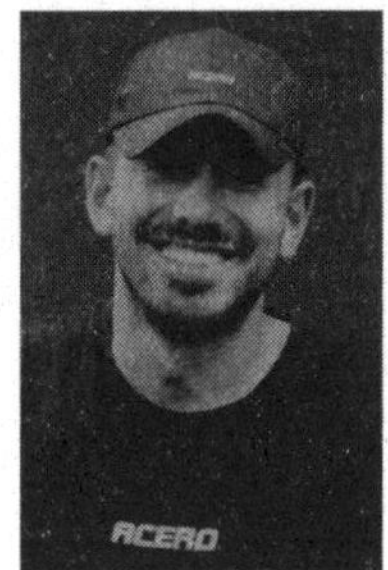

Jono Castano is a personal trainer and the inhouse trainer at *Men's Health Magazine*. He has 849k+ followers on Instagram (86% of which are located in Australia), and his celebrity clients range from Michael Clarke and Dustin Martin to Sir Richard Branson.

IT STARTS TODAY

IT STARTS TODAY

JONO CASTANO

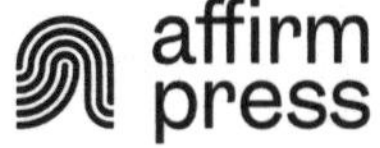

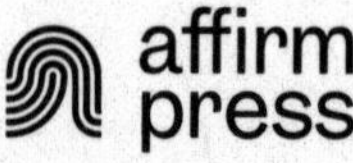

First published by Affirm Press in 2024
Bunurong/Boon Wurrung Country
28 Thistlethwaite Street
South Melbourne VIC 3205
affirmpress.com.au

10 9 8 7 6 5 4 3 2 1

This work was made on the unceded land of the Bunurong/Boon Wurrung peoples of the Kulin Nation. Affirm Press pays respect to their elders past and present.

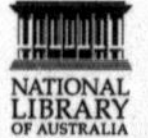

A catalogue record for this book is available from the National Library of Australia

ISBN: 9781922992215 (paperback)

Cover design by Luke Causby/Blue Cork © Affirm Press
Cover photo from David Swift Photography on Newspix, 2019
Typeset in 12.25/19 pt Sabon LT Pro by Post Pre-press Group, Brisbane
Proudly printed and bound in Australia by McPherson's Printing Group

CONTENTS

INTRODUCTION

You've got big plans and saintly intentions. This time you're finally going to get in serious shape. You're determined to get stronger and fitter by sticking to your exercise regimen and making it to every session come rain or shine. While you're at it, you're going to get healthier, too – clean up your diet, curb the mid-week boozing and make a concerted effort to get more sleep.

You're going to start soon, too. You just need to settle on a date as the launch pad to this new improved you. The one who's going to be leaner, kinder, sexier and far less grumpy first thing in the morning. Maybe you'll start on New Year's Day or after your birthday in a couple of months' time? Maybe you'll wait until things aren't so crazy at work? Or when your youngest kid starts school? Or when it's less hot (or less cold)? Or when your renovation is finally done? Or when your back stops aching? Or when that new gym opens down the street?

ENOUGH ALREADY. IT STARTS TODAY.

I know what you're thinking: you don't know where to begin. You need to find a personal trainer to help you along. Plus, shouldn't you really empty the freezer of all those party pies and mint-choc-chip Cornettos? My advice is don't delay. If you've resolved to make a change in your life, the best thing you can do is just get going. Don't over-think it, just start.

One thing I've learned after helping thousands of people get into the best shape of their lives is that attitude follows behaviour, not the other way around. Never underestimate the power of momentum. It's like pushing a car – once you overcome that initial sticking point of inertia, it'll often begin rolling along with surprising ease.

You might be thinking it's not a good time. Your horrible boss just buried you alive under an avalanche of deadlines and you need to slog your way out. Your landlord just put your rent up (again) and you have to find a new place to live. Your toddler is teething and proving a real handful at the moment so it's hard for you to escape to the gym. I get it. Those are all legitimate stressors. But the truth is, there will always be some form of obstacle in your path. Real life is messy and unpredictable and delights in setting malicious booby-traps for your carefully laid plans. Just as people say there's never a perfect time to have a baby, the perfect conditions for you to get fit will never arise. Instead, what you must learn to do is integrate your health and wellness goals into the howling chaos that is the shit-storm of your daily life.

Maybe you don't feel sufficiently motivated at this precise moment. You don't want to set yourself up for failure by jumping the gun and then doing a half-arsed job. The problem is that inspiration alone will never get you fit. There'll always be days when it's cold outside or you're feeling too tired or sore or stressed or busy or depressed. Your willpower alone will never match the size of the task ahead.

YOU JUST HAVE TO GET STARTED AND COMMIT.

Procrastination is a complex adversary. It's often linked to a deeper issue, whether that's anxiety, lack of confidence or perfectionism. Yet whatever the root cause, it can paralyse you from leading the sort of life you want to lead. Ultimately, procrastination is vertical gravity – it keeps you glued to the same dismal spot when you need to be moving forward to get your hands on the good stuff. Procrastination's most damaging effect is that it steals your time, robbing days, weeks and years from your life. That's an issue because time is the most valuable commodity you have.

I've trained successful people from many walks of life – from Richard Branson and Rita Ora to Alexander Volkanovski. One thing I've noticed these people have in common is they understand the true value of their time. Having made it big, their daily schedules are crazier than ever. That means their time is scarcer and therefore more valuable. And that is why they don't procrastinate – their time is too precious to waste.

You've probably heard the old joke: 'My mother always told me I wouldn't amount to anything because I procrastinate. I said, "Just wait …"' Unfortunately, the mum in question may have had a point. Studies have found that procrastination has a negative impact on both body and mind with the habit linked to great levels of stress, anxiety, depression, sleep deprivation and poorer work performance, too.[1] In short, it's bad news all around.

If you've picked up this book, you presumably want to supercharge some area of your health and wellness. Good on you. The mere fact that you're reading this suggests that you're open to making changes. My advice is to start backing those great intentions with actions right away. Sure, you may refine your habits, tweak your diet or alter your training as you go along. But as soon as you embark on this odyssey of self-optimisation, you'll be making positive changes and starting to form better habits and routines that you can build upon. Chances are you'll enjoy some early wins that will propel you forward with extra motivation under your belt. Keep going and you'll start to feel better about yourself and even more in control. A better future really could await if you're willing to take the chance and get with the program. And you know what the really exciting part is? It starts today.

HE WHO WISHES MISSES

Remember the story of Aladdin? To recap: a young, impoverished guy manages to get his hands on a magical lamp. When he accidentally rubs it, a genie appears. This genie can make Aladdin's every wish come true. Our boy consequently winds up with unimaginable wealth, a magnificent palace and the hand in marriage of the sultan's absolute knockout of a daughter. Possibly a magic carpet or two as well. But here's the thing: you don't need a supernatural lamp to get what you want in life. All you need to do is take action.

I live by the sincere belief that he who wishes misses. That's because a wish is merely an empty hope that you'll get something or that a specific occurrence will happen to you. It's a hankering devoid of any real substance. People wish that they could become successful entrepreneurs. They wish for a life partner with whom they'll live happily ever after. They wish they could lose 20 kilograms. The problem is that a wish is just a dream for the future. Sure, it may be deeply heartfelt – you may yearn for that one thing so much that it makes your chest ache. But it remains a dream nonetheless. And the sad truth is that dreams tend to be flimsy, ephemeral things that aren't very reliable. They don't stand up to the unsympathetic glare of real life that deals in hard facts and tangible actions.

IF YOU REALLY WANT TO MAKE SOMETHING HAPPEN YOU HAVE TO *MAKE SOMETHING HAPPEN.*

Wishing alone is never enough. Instead, you need to take that dream and put some meat on its (wish)bones. The reason you don't need that genie is that you have the power within yourself to realise your ambitions. You just need to find a way to harness it. The way to do that is to find your sense of purpose and an overarching plan that maps out how you're going to achieve your goal; to break it down into concrete steps and manageable micro-goals that'll lead you along the way. Pulling that plan together is the first step. Then you're going to roll up your sleeves and attack it with everything you've got.

Seriously though, enough with this wishing business. You really want to be a successful entrepreneur? Start off by developing a business plan, becoming an expert in your chosen field, finding a mentor and networking with serious purpose and intent. You want to find that life partner? Give yourself the best possible shot and start hanging out in places where that person may lurk, whether that's dating apps, coffee shops, dog parks or pubs – Cupid's arrow won't hit you when you're sitting on your couch in your tracky dacks halfway through a family sized pack of Cheezels. You really want to lose weight? Take a good hard look at your daily nutrition and dedicate yourself to an exercise plan (and stick to it).

Listen, I'm not going to bullshit you: this isn't a foolproof plan. Life is complicated and there are no certainties. Ultimately your success will come down to you. But to give yourself any chance you need to back your dreams up with serious action. As Michael Jordan once put it, 'Some people want it to happen, some wish it would happen, others make it happen.' That make-it-happen category is where you're going to be.

FIND YOUR PURPOSE

You planned to go for a run after work, except it looks like it might rain and you don't want to get soaked. Plus, it's been a really stressful day – you've got a massive deadline looming on Friday and you weren't very productive in the office because that planning meeting ran way overtime. Frankly, you feel bloody exhausted, too. You had a horrible night's sleep. You woke up at 3am and stared at the ceiling, worrying about all sorts of things from your mortgage payments to that upcoming deadline and that weird rash you've got on your leg. So maybe you won't go for that run today after all. There's just far too much going on.

I mention this imaginary scenario because it's exactly the sort of situation that you'll find yourself in over and over again. Life is relentless and particularly unkind when it comes to sabotaging your fitness goals. There are so many daily curveballs that can suddenly bounce up, knock you in the teeth (ouch!), make you spill your coffee (aargh!) and, most importantly, stop you following through with your good intentions.

The real issue for most people isn't *starting* a health and fitness regimen, but sticking with it – showing up again and again, week after week to train consistently and follow the plan right through to completion. The challenge is finding the motivation to persist, even on those days when you're dog-tired and stressed out of your mind. If you don't, it will stop you from reaching your target, whatever that may be.

What you need to avoid succumbing to that pressure is to find something that's much bigger than all those annoyances and distractions. In fact, it's so much greater that it dwarfs those trivial complications and puts them into perspective, overshadowing them to the point where they become piddly and insignificant in comparison. What you need is to find your purpose.

As a personal trainer who's worked with dozens of celebrities over the years to help them with dramatic transformations, people often ask me how they can imitate these high-profile journeys, wanting to lose up to 20 kilograms in the process. While it's true that I usually train these celebrities over a long period of time and help them along on their journey, the crucial breakthrough, in fact, happens before we even meet. When people seek me out, they've often already found their purpose. They don't want to start training merely to lose a set number of kilos. They aren't exercising to fit into a certain clothing size. They have simply reached a point in their life where they've decided to take control of their wellbeing.

Sometimes there are momentous reasons why people commit to getting healthier, too, such as improving their quality of life and/or living longer, whether that's for the sake of themselves or their children. A healthier lifestyle helps to protect us against serious health problems, such as diabetes, high blood pressure and heart disease.

A purpose like this is what keeps my long-term clients strong and committed in the weeks and months ahead. That yearning to be better ensures that they stick to their training plan even when they have to work long hours or are faced with temptation.

IF YOU'RE SERIOUS ABOUT MAKING BIG CHANGES TO YOUR OWN HEALTH AND FITNESS, YOU NEED TO FIND YOUR PURPOSE.

Your purpose must become your guiding star as you slog through the mountain of additional responsibilities all of us face – work, family, parenthood or whatever other eye-watering craziness that you happen to have on your plate. Your purpose needs to be strong enough that it can withstand being buffeted on all sides by those other powerful forces. When it comes to finding your purpose, you have to think *big*.

Ask most people why they're training and they'll struggle to identify a strong purpose. They might talk about wanting to fit into their old jeans or shape up ahead of a beach holiday. There's nothing fundamentally wrong with those reasons, but I'm not sure a pair of jeans is enough to inspire you to get into your gym kit when your alarm goes off at 5am and it's freezing outside and you're slightly hungover from the night before. You're going to need heroic reserves of energy, determination and focus to keep on trucking through the weeks and months that lie ahead. Your purpose must be meaningful enough to sustain and inspire you to keep on going. As Friedrich Nietzsche (a big fan of high intensity interval training, I believe) once said: 'He who has a why to live for can bear almost any how.'

So how do you find your purpose? When I'm working with a client I start by getting them to answer a series of questions.

THE FIRST IS, 'WHO AM I?'

The idea here is to define who you are in terms of your current life roles. That extends to your family (you might, for example, be a mother, husband, sister, son and so on) and also to your working and social life. This should help you to see your responsibilities from every angle. The question also pertains to your physical and emotional life. I'd want you to describe your physical scenario – your current weight, health and fitness – and whether you're happy with your present situation. You might, for example, want to get back in shape to feel more confident at work or to boost your self-esteem after a break-up. But I'd also want you to reflect on your emotional position – whether you're happy or dissatisfied in any key areas of life. This question is really about taking a snapshot of your ground zero and considering where you're at right now.

THE SECOND QUESTION IS, 'WHAT DO I STAND FOR?'

You might think of yourself as a hardworking provider or a good team player. You might be a great listener or a social connector that brings people together. This question is about defining the values that you embrace, the principles that guide your behaviour and the character traits that define your personality (or that you want people to associate with you).

THE FINAL QUESTION IS 'WHAT DO I WANT TO BE?'

How do you want to operate in life? How do you want to present yourself? How do you want to treat other people? Perhaps you want to become more patient with your children, or less stressed at work. You might want to become someone with a healthier relationship with food or drink or recreational drugs. It's another big question that's worth approaching from multiple angles – your career, your family life, your relationships and your mental and physical health. If you could take control of each of these elements, how would you ideally change them?

These questions are designed to get you thinking about the bigger picture for your life and hopefully prompt you to find your deeper purpose. I know this might all sound a bit fluffy, but I'm hammering this message home because it's actually rooted in hard-headed practicality. My job as a personal trainer is to help people achieve the results they crave. And of all the people I've trained over the years, those who've been the most successful in their quests are those who've managed to identify their bigger purpose.

I trained one guy, for example, who'd become a dad on the cusp of turning 50. His purpose was to get fit so he could play with his young kids with more energy and stay limber enough to be able to go surfing with them when they reached their teens. Another lady I worked with found she had really high visceral fat levels. The purpose behind her training was to improve her health and lower her risk of having a heart attack. I also know tons of people who train as a proactive measure for their mental equilibrium and use it as part of their strategy to keep depression at bay.

Those are all big, meaty examples of purpose. You need to unlock a similar source of deep motivation that will push you through those moments of self-doubt and hesitation, lift you above all those niggling inconveniences and ensure that you lace up your sneakers to go for that run. (Even though it has actually now started to rain.)

A BRIEF HISTORY OF **JONO CASTANO**

It was 2014. I'd just scored my very first job as a personal trainer with Virgin Active. The gym had a shiny new premises opening in Sydney's inner suburb of Zetland. To commemorate the occasion we were getting a special visit from the man himself, Richard Branson.

Few other businesspeople in the world are on Richard Branson's level. It was like getting a visit from a rock star. Everyone was so excited and started crowding around him. I remember being surprised by how lean and energetic he looked for his age as he walked through the gym, smiling for photos and shaking hands. But that was the only impression

I really had, because I never got anywhere near him. After all, I was just a rookie trainer; the gym's management reserved Branson's press-the-flesh time for the most senior staff and key clientele. I didn't even get to speak to the man and, while I understood the reasoning, I remember going home that night feeling slightly deflated.

Seven years later life had changed dramatically. I'd built my own successful gym, Acero, and become Australia's biggest celebrity trainer in the process. I was holidaying in Miami when, out of the blue, I got a message from Richard Branson's team asking whether I'd consider coming to train him on his private yacht. Obviously, I jumped at the chance.

That was a pinch-yourself moment because it demonstrated how far I'd come in the space of seven years. Admittedly, it hadn't been a seamless ascent - I made plenty of mistakes in both my private and professional life during that time, and have since. Somehow, though, I've managed to battle my way through. Acero is now performing strongly enough that we're looking to expand to Los Angeles, while our app, Acero Drip, is making our training accessible to people all over the world. To give you some insight into my journey, here's a brief history of my 32 years on the planet.

MY ORIGIN STORY

I grew up in Colombia in a small town called La Virginia that's situated in a landlocked region in the central west. Out there, life for most people is tough and, by Western standards, the living conditions remain fairly primitive. Growing up we never had hot running water, and people still used carts and horses as one of the main forms of transport. Our family never really had any money, but as kids you don't notice those things. I had a happy childhood growing up with my parents and two older brothers, Damian and Mauricio.

My father yearned to build a better life for the family. Like most of the men in La Virginia, he supported us by working in the surrounding fields cutting sugarcane. My dad is an insanely hard worker who you'll never hear complain, but toiling in the sugarcane fields is hot, backbreaking labour. Each day he'd leave for work in the early hours, sometimes around 3am before the sun became too intense. Dad and his workmates would then slave away all day, their hands getting calloused from their machetes and their feet bitten by caterpillars and scorpions. It was a physically demanding job where, however hard you worked, you'd still only be making the bare minimum to keep your family alive.

Yet it wasn't just the poverty that prompted my dad to dream of escape. Colombia is a dangerous country, too, where violence is part of life. I remember as a kid seeing someone shot in one of the local streets. The issue of safety hit home for our family in a tragic way when my oldest brother was killed in a road accident. Mauricio was only six years old and was sitting on the back of a motorcycle. As it went over a bridge, the motorcycle suddenly hit a pothole and Mauricio was flung off the back of the bike into oncoming traffic.

I was still a baby when that accident happened - too young to register the tragedy. But Mauricio's death devastated the family. It was heartbreaking for my parents to lose their oldest child in such a senseless way. The death of his son made my dad even more determined to get the family out of Colombia. He knew that if we stayed there, the family would be stuck in the poverty cycle as he worked his life away in the sugarcane fields for $100 a month. His biggest fear was that, if we remained, the life options for me and my brother would be exactly the same as they were for him. If you're a family of modest means in rural Colombia, and you want to live comfortably and remain on the right side of the law, your opportunities are extremely limited.

My father became obsessed with trying to forge a better future for his family. To achieve this, he believed, we had to get away. First, Dad tried to get a visa to live in Miami - where most Colombians try to go - but he was rejected. Then he tried to get a visa for the UK, but once again he was knocked back. After that failure, Dad set his sights on Australia. Finally he got a tourist visa and opted to go off on his own with the plan of bringing the rest of the family over as soon as he could - he couldn't afford plane tickets for the four of us on a sugarcane worker's paltry wage. Looking back, it was a huge decision for my father. He didn't speak any English and had almost no money - all he had in Sydney was one friend. It must have taken so much courage to make that move, not to mention a fair amount of desperation.

I didn't see my father for two years. He was forced to spend six months in an Australian detention centre and, when he eventually got out, he was determined to earn money any way he could. Getting a job wasn't easy since he didn't speak English, but he took whatever jobs presented themselves - from cleaning work to construction. Armed with his work ethic and the desire to reunite with his family, Dad grafted tirelessly. It must have been a fairly joyless existence: he lived on a super-tight budget saving every cent that he could. But that was what he had to do to get his family back together.

THE FAMILY REUNITED

The rest of us eventually moved to Australia in 1998 when I was seven years old. We settled in Mascot, not far from

Sydney Airport. What I remember most from those early years in Australia is that my parents were constantly working, working, working. They were grateful for the opportunity to earn money; they both took cleaning jobs and ground away every single day. Even when my mum was home, she was trying to make extra cash by turning our garage into a little corner store selling chocolates and chips. My parents' entire life at that time was dedicated to building the foundation that would give our family a more stable future.

The language barrier was the hardest thing for me. At first I couldn't speak any English at all so I struggled at school. My lack of fluency in English made life in the playground hard. Young kids always notice anyone who's different, so I copped a fair bit of teasing and bullying. Looking back it wasn't the easiest time, but luckily I had one outlet that made my life bearable.

When we arrived in Australia my parents put me straight into a local soccer team: the Mascot Kings. I may have struggled to express myself at school due to my lack of English, but one area where I could excel was on the pitch. Soccer became my escape, the safe place where I felt comfortable. Putting on my boots and walking onto the field felt like home. Better still, because I had some natural talent, I instantly got a lot of praise that boosted my confidence at a time when I needed it the most. All I wanted to do was to play soccer every single day. I dedicated my life to it, practising for hours and hours every night after school, kicking a ball against the wall or playing with my brother. Then I'd play matches on the weekends, before coming home to play even more soccer.

When I was nine we moved to a suburb called Meadowbank. I joined a team called the West Ryde Rovers and, after a while, I began to play for the junior teams of the Marconi Stallions - one of the best clubs in the National Soccer League. Over time, I became a decent centre midfielder, a box-to-box player who was comfortable with both feet and willing to run all day. At 13 I was chosen to play in the New South Wales squad for a tournament between all the states and territories. I was named player of the tournament and started to dream of becoming a professional.

From then on I fixated on that ambition. Later that year I had the chance to train in England at the West Ham United Academy. As a soccer-mad teenager I was living the dream and the step-up in pressure to perform quality didn't faze me either. Unfortunately I was only on a three-month tourist visa, so when that came to an end, I had to go home. I honestly believe that if I'd had a European passport, West Ham would probably have signed me up. That experience only sharpened my hunger to succeed.

I wound up going to school at Westfields Sports High School. Based in Sydney's western suburbs, the school is pretty much dedicated to sport; you do the bare minimum of academic subjects to get by. Former pupils include Michael Clarke, Harry Kewell, Usman Khawaja and Israel Folau - the list goes on and on. The quality of soccer players when I was there was super high - Aaron Mooy and Mathew Ryan were in my year and both went on to play for the Socceroos and in top European leagues. At that stage I could hold my own in that company and I started plotting my career.

So began a crazy few years in which I travelled the world looking to make it as a professional soccer player. First I went to Colombia, where I joined Academia Fútbol Club in Bogotá. It was a second-division team and I was playing for the reserves and training with the first team. Suddenly I was living and breathing soccer 24 hours a day. I'd wake up, eat, train and then repeat the process, over and over again. I felt like I was finally en route to my dream.

I was desperate to play in Europe: that's where you can really make a name for yourself. Belgium is a well-trodden pathway for Australian players because it's easier to get a visa, so I jumped at the chance to play for a small club called RRFC Montegnée in Liège. I was there for a season, but my agent kept telling me I had a good chance in the A-League back in Australia. So I came back home and tried out with the Newcastle Jets, but was passed over - at which point my career became increasingly exotic. I played for a season in Singapore and a season in Indonesia. Basically, I'd play for a season and then go back home, because I'd always wanted to play in the big leagues and saw how difficult it was to be spotted at one of the minor clubs in a far-flung league. Every time I went abroad and it didn't work out, I realised that my options were narrowing and my dream of becoming a successful professional player was fading. At the same time, though, I didn't know anything else but soccer.

One of the worst experiences I had during that time was when my agent said he'd organised a trial for me with a club in Israel. At that stage I was working at Coles stacking shelves and was desperate for any opportunity. I travelled all the way over to Israel, turned up at the training grounds and explained I was there for the trial. The coach just looked at me blankly. 'I don't know who you are, I've never heard of your agent and I've never spoken to anyone about you,' he said. He wouldn't even let me stay for a trial, so I had no choice but to go all the way back home. Bear in mind I was still barely 20 years old, so those sorts of knockbacks were brutal. But while I did get upset, those experiences also toughened me up and gave me a thicker skin.

The hardest part for me was that my parents helped to fund a lot of those trips. The way it worked is that you'd pay your own way over to these countries and you'd only be reimbursed if the club decided to sign you up. By this stage my dad was working as a welder. I saw how hard my parents were working to try to facilitate my dream. I was acutely conscious of their sacrifice and desperate to make it worthwhile. When I was trialling at a new club I felt so much pressure to play well. It became really intense. Sport is a meritocracy, but there's an element of luck involved when you're trying to establish yourself, too. Sometimes you might have the best game of your life and score a hat-trick, only to find out the relevant coach wasn't watching; then, inevitably, that coach would turn up when you'd just missed an open goal. I kept hustling and continued to travel for opportunities, but after a while the rejections took their toll. It's hard when you're a young guy, living away from home in a country where you don't speak the language and things aren't going well for you on the pitch. The negativity soon begins to mount. The final straw came after I did a trial for a team in Armenia of all places. I felt I'd given a good account of myself after playing well in the preseason tour to Turkey and Anatolia. Suddenly, however, the club changed its policy and decided it wouldn't sign any new players that year. That was when I decided it was time to come home.

THE FIRST SPARKS OF A NEW CAREER

Back in Sydney I was still playing state soccer while trying to support myself in other ways, too. I took on a retail job at Adidas but was also trying to nut out what I was going to do long-term now that my lifelong dream of becoming a professional soccer player was over. I had a girlfriend, Amy, whose parents suggested I join the police force. I was so lost at the time that I figured, well, why not? I went through the application process and was about to go to the academy in Canberra, but I never went through with it - for the simple reason that I'd discovered personal training in the meantime.

Years of playing soccer had given me a real interest in physical performance - how to train to build speed, strength and power. So I did a personal trainer course and started doing private sessions with a handful of clients before and after work. I loved it right from the beginning. What I got out of personal training was a sense of the teamwork and camaraderie that I'd previously enjoyed from playing soccer. I liked the connection that I built with each individual, the journey that we went on together and the positive effect I could have on someone's life. Exercise can be such a powerful tool. Not only was I helping people become fitter and stronger, but I often saw a change in them mentally, too. I usually find it quite easy to strike up a personal connection with a client and that's mainly, I suspect, because I have a genuine interest in their lives and motivations. I want to understand why they haven't reached their goals in the past and figure out how we can work together to change that.

Being a personal trainer is all about those interpersonal relationships and I benefited from them, too. Early on, when a client would thank me for a great session, I'd get such a buzz out of that compliment. Deep down, I now realise, my confidence was still pretty low because I'd failed to make a career out of soccer. Working as a personal trainer gave me the sense of personal affirmation that I needed. That was when I ditched my plan to become a cop and decided to build a career as a personal trainer instead. Soon after making that life-changing decision I moved from Sydney's west to the Eastern Suburbs - I felt that was where the opportunities for a successful personal trainer would be. If I was going to do this I wanted to go all-in.

Over the next decade I worked for a bunch of gyms from Virgin Active to Fitness First to a variety of private spaces. I progressed fairly quickly. My work ethic and drive helped me in that regard. Nothing came easy to me at first; I was even turned down for my first job at Virgin Active, twice! I kept putting myself forward until my persistence eventually convinced the company to give me a shot. Once my foot was in that door I was determined to capitalise on the opportunity by working harder than anyone else. Virgin Active had a leaderboard that kept track of how many sessions each trainer across the world was doing. In my first year I became the number-one trainer in Virgin Active's global system. I was doing up to 84 sessions with clients every single week. I was prepared to grind harder than everyone else.

That work ethic, I believe, came from my upbringing. I remembered how hard it was for people to make a living back in Colombia and the work they'd endure to feed their families. For years I'd watched my parents take on whatever overtime they could if it meant they'd earn a bit of extra cash. Don't get me wrong - sometimes when my alarm goes off at 4am so I can get to my first training session I do wish I could spend an extra hour in bed. But I also recognise my good fortune. It's not like I'm having to break rocks in the burning sun to earn my keep.

Then again, a lot of personal trainers have the right attitude and are prepared to work hard. Another reason I believe my career accelerated so quickly is that I was dead set on taking full responsibility for its trajectory. I didn't want my success to depend on other people. When I was playing soccer there were so many random external factors that I couldn't influence. If I made a good run, would my teammate spot it? Would the right scout be watching me at the right time on the right day? Would the club politics sanction a new signing? I wanted ownership of my future. I wanted to take control of my destiny and not be reliant on others' whims. If personal training was to be my career path, I wanted to take charge of how it unfolded.

The way it usually works for personal trainers is that you pay your gym a form of rent to operate using their facilities, and then you keep the money your clients pay you. The onus is on you to sign up as many new clients as you can. But the question is, how do you stand out from the crowd? These days there are so many amazing personal trainers out there - people who are personable, committed and knowledgeable. It's a massively competitive world, and when you're starting out, it's hard to distinguish yourself and grow your clientele. As Mark Bouris said when he interviewed me for his podcast, *The Mentor with Mark Bouris*: 'I reckon personal training is one of the hardest gigs in the world.'

A SPRINKLE OF STARDUST

Social media was the game changer for me. I jumped on it in the early days when a lot of other trainers were still suspicious of the format. I viewed it as a way to market what I was doing for free. I needed to find a way to reach more clients - I was still a young trainer and didn't have the network more established people enjoyed. I used Instagram as a platform to showcase my personality, my training and the results that I could deliver to my clients. I was also willing to take a risk and be a bit more playful with my content, such as posting a photo of myself wearing a skimpy pair of budgie smugglers.

I appreciate that none of that sounds particularly ground-breaking now; but, back then, a lot of personal trainers still portrayed themselves as stern-faced drill-sergeant types whose schtick was barking orders while trying to look tough. I decided to take a more lighthearted path. I wanted to make sure I seemed approachable. I was quite happy to take the piss out of myself on social media because that was a more authentic reflection of how I lived my life. Back in 2014, that way of doing things was still new and I got a lot of criticism. I remember a manager at Virgin Active telling me, 'What are you doing on Instagram? You can't be posting this sort of stuff!' Luckily my experience in soccer had made me pretty resilient to personal criticism. Amy, my soon-to-be wife, was so important at that stage of my life, too. When I was copping flak about my social posts and getting all these snarky comments, she supported me all the way. 'Jono, just keep going,' she'd say. 'These people mean nothing to you.'

And I did keep going because I could see that my content resonated. My Instagram audience was growing. Having built a credible following, I then decided to leverage it in a different way. By this stage I was increasingly in demand as a personal trainer, but I knew that if I could win some high-profile clients it could change the perception of my entire business. Essentially I needed to sprinkle a little star-dust over my brand. At the same time, as a kid from Sydney's west, I didn't have an address book full of showbiz contacts to call on. I decided to use Instagram to start reaching out to people with a public profile and a big social media presence. Effectively I was cold-calling them by sending them direct messages, but what did I have to lose?

The first person I contacted was Matty J (Matt Johnson) who was about to be the main man on *The Bachelor* in 2017. I just pinged him a DM and offered to train him for free. It was a win-win scenario. Matty was securing free access to an experienced trainer and decent gym facilities. What was in it for me? While I had no expectation that Matty would post anything about his training, I suspected that if I did a good job and got him into killer shape there was a chance of getting some exposure. Not only did that plan work - Matty got absolutely shredded - but the *Daily Mail Australia* picked up the story and interviewed me about the transformation, describing me as a 'former soccer player turned fitness guru'.[2]

I repeated the process again and again. I trained a few people from *Australian Idol* including Jessica Mauboy, Casey Donovan and Paulini. I trained pop duo the Veronicas and a few other reality TV stars, such as Timomatic, who were enjoying their moment in the sun. Again, these were all mutually beneficial relationships. There's a lot of pressure for public figures to stay in shape and I was helping them achieve that for free.

The strategy quickly built momentum and bigger names soon began to seek me out. Celebrity clients recommended me to their high-profile friends - for example, I trained the actor Hugh Sheridan. Soon I found myself training singers such as Rita Ora, actors such as *Home and Away*'s Pia Miller and Lincoln Lewis, sportspeople such as Michael Clarke and Alex Volkanovski and businesspeople such as Richard Branson and Roxy Jacenko. The media coverage grew. I became the transformation coach for *Men's Health* Australia. I was being asked to contribute expert articles to various media outlets and being invited onto *Sunrise* to talk about my training programs. Suddenly, the business that I'd formed with Amy was flying. We opened our own gym, Acero, in Kensington, Sydney.

I recently worked out that I've completed almost 50,000 training sessions with clients since 2014. That's allowed me to observe a huge number of real-life case studies and figure out what works and what doesn't. Through that process, I've gleaned the most effective strategies to help people get the results they crave without having to lead joyless lives of self-denial. I've found there isn't one single secret to guarantee success. But there are five interlocking pillars that can help you make lasting and dramatic changes to your health and fitness: your mindset, how you exercise, your nutrition, your sleep and achieving a true sense of balance. This book will unpack those pillars in depth, empowering you to become healthier, happier and even more comfortable in your own skin.

PILLAR 1

MINDSET

If you want to get fitter, leaner or stronger, there's one part of your body that you simply cannot afford to neglect. It's not your arms or your core. It's not your legs or your back. The most important muscle - the one that will make the crucial difference between success and failure - is situated right between your ears.

Pedants might point out that the brain isn't technically a muscle, a point that I will reluctantly concede (because it's true). But it's still the all-important element in any health and fitness journey. That's because your mind is what ultimately calls the shots on your behaviour. It can steer you in the right direction and ensure you get enough sleep, exercise and good nutrition, or it can sabotage your intentions and send you spiralling down a less helpful path – fast food, booze and god only knows what else. Forging the right mindset is the critical factor in training consistently and looking after yourself. Once you've found your guiding purpose, which we talked about earlier in the book, you need to cultivate a favourable environment for it to thrive. To use a gardening analogy, if your purpose is like a young sapling, your mindset is the garden that must offer the right conditions for the tree to grow healthy and strong.

RETHINK YOUR LIMITATIONS

Training Michael Clarke was a privilege. I used to watch Australia's former Test skipper at the crease. He was such a masterful batsman due to his immaculate timing and ability to play the ball on the rise. But as he stroked the ball around the oval, you'd never guess that he was battling chronic pain. Things hadn't improved in that department since he retired from the game, either. When Michael came to train with me for a 12-week transformation for *Men's Health*, his back was causing him all sorts of grief. With three degenerative discs in his lower back, he admitted there were times when the stiffness and discomfort got so intense that he couldn't even bend down to put on his shoes and socks. Michael was therefore understandably worried that his back would make many exercises impossible.

Now, training with me isn't a walk in the park – it's more akin to a succession of back-to-back sprints supersetted with push-ups! While I respected that Michael had a genuine issue to manage, I didn't want it to hold him back mentally. I was concerned that Michael might not fully commit due to his back problems, or would use his condition as a get-out clause to avoid going full pelt. That's why, at the outset, we came up with a deal. Michael and I agreed that he would attempt whatever exercises I prescribed him. If it turned out he couldn't physically manage them because of his back, that was totally fine. But he had to be open to the challenge.

To be honest, it turned out there was hardly anything that Michael couldn't do. He liked to be tested and worked super hard in the gym, getting through a huge workload that boosted his strength and agility. At the end of the challenge, Michael admitted that he looked and felt better than he ever had when he was a professional athlete.

It would've been so easy for Michael to have psyched himself out right from the beginning. He could've used his back problems as a white flag to wave whenever the workouts got tough. Instead he refused to let his physical limitations define his capabilities or limit his potential. That was so important because it meant that he didn't lower the ceiling for what he could achieve.

HOW DOES THIS RELATE TO YOU?

Sit down for a minute and write down a list of your realistic capabilities when it comes to your physical potential. Could you ever run a marathon? Stand on your head? Bang out ten pull-ups with strict form? Now rip up the list and start again. Because I'm pretty sure that whatever you wrote down on that list was horribly undercooked. In fact, I suspect that it failed to even begin to do justice to what you could really do.

I say that having regularly watched people in my gym achieve mind-blowing progressions in strength and fitness that far outstrip their expectations. Take Richard, a guy in his late fifties who I currently train. At first he was out of condition and well above his ideal healthy weight. Even after doing ten standing push-ups off the wall, he'd have to rest for three minutes to lower his heart rate back to a safe level. Now, six months later, he's banging out 30 push-ups on a pair of YBells with ease. Richard can't believe how far he's come. But I can, because I've seen it happen time and again.

The truth is that we're capable of so much more than what we know. Our biggest adversary usually exists in our own minds. In other words, the barriers that stop us tend to be psychological, not physiological. These limitations are self-enforcing, too. If you convince yourself you can't do something, you never will.

THE FOUR-MINUTE MILE

Our own psychological barriers also tend to prove contagious to other people. One of the most famous examples of this is the four-minute mile. For many years, the idea of running a mile in under four minutes was dismissed as a physical impossibility. The idea was spoken of in hushed tones as the athletic holy grail, a form of sporting Valhalla that was too fanciful to seriously consider.

In 1935 Brutus Hamilton, a highly respected track coach at the University of California, set out to determine the limit of physical performance in a variety of athletic pursuits. To do this in a scientific manner, Hamilton enlisted a team of Finnish physicists to create graphs on human energy, expectancy and fatigue. Informed by this exhaustive list of facts and figures, Hamilton issued a list of the 'ultimates of human effort' for various track and field pursuits that ranged from the pole vault to the shot-put. The fastest a man could run a mile, Hamilton believed, was four minutes and 1.66 seconds.

Luckily, not everyone agreed with this scientific verdict. In England, amateur runner and young medical student Roger Bannister, saw the four-minute mile as 'a challenge of the human spirit'. For eight years, Bannister trained week after week to the point of collapse. Using his medical knowledge he measured his lactic acid levels and often trained with an oxygen mask to give his muscles extra fuel. Bannister overhauled his running style, refining it to achieve the maximum energy-to-speed ratio. He even commissioned a cobbler to make him a special pair of race shoes that were 50 per cent lighter than his previous pair. These painstaking efforts ultimately paid off on 6 May 1954 when Bannister achieved the unattainable and ran the mile in three minutes 59.4 seconds, collapsing across the finish line. Bannister later wrote that he felt 'like an exploded flashlight'.

The most remarkable impact of this feat was its knock-on effect. People had attempted to run a sub-four-minute mile for decades without success. Bannister managing to do it changed the collective mindset. Suddenly, people attempted the distance propelled by a renewed sense of possibility and belief. A mere 46 days after Bannister's achievement, Australian John Landy broke the record, running the mile in three minutes 58 seconds. Barely a year later, three more runners managed to complete a sub-four-minute mile in a single race.

During that period there'd been no quantum leap in human evolution. Our genetic biology had not abruptly changed. The only thing that had shifted was the prevailing mindset on what was possible.

By breaking the four-minute barrier, Bannister had single-handedly expanded the preconceived boundaries of endurance. More importantly, though, he'd smashed the dominant belief to pieces. Bannister's secret was realising that mental strength and resolve are ultimately the deciding factors in athletic performance. As he later wrote: 'It is the brain, not the heart or lungs, that is the critical organ.'

THE TAKE-HOME MESSAGE FROM BANNISTER'S FOUR-MINUTE MILE IS THAT YOUR CAPABILITIES ARE OFTEN FAR GREATER THAN YOU BELIEVE.

Sometimes you do need someone to show you the way – whether that's a personal trainer, coach or training partner. But you also need to put yourself in a state where you'll be receptive to their information or example. If you have a closed mind or a pessimistic outlook, those positive messages will bounce off and never have any chance to permeate.

If you're training towards a particular goal, you have to stay aware of your mental state and police your thought processes for negativity. Sometimes you may develop a belief that's not necessarily true, or a nagging idea that's not particularly helpful might percolate. At such times, you need to step back and objectively dissect the logical basis of that notion that's pinballing through your head. Is it really accurate? Or is it a self-defeating assumption?

A good way of ascertaining the truth is to ask yourself the question:

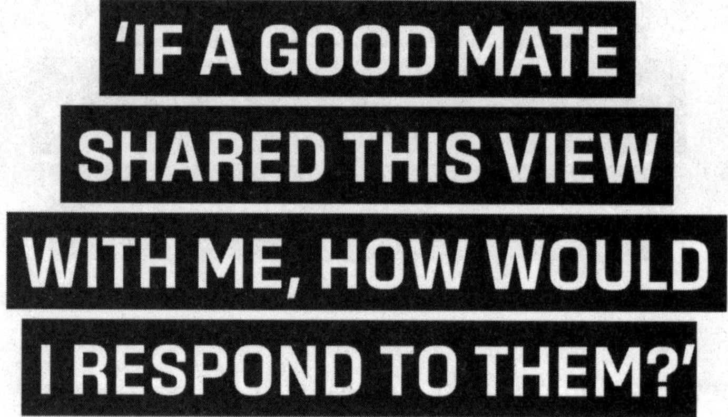

Most of the time, I expect, your response would provide them with a sense of perspective, kindness and comfort. Yet our self-talk is often pointlessly negative and harsh. Make a conscious effort to hit the mute button on this inner critic. Your mind can be the ultimate trash-talker when it comes to your potential. Many of these rogue thoughts simply don't deserve space in your head.

GET COMFORTABLE BEING UNCOMFORTABLE

One of the most inspiring recent examples of redefining physical potential came in the form of a 23-year-old electrician with a bleach-blond mullet. I'm talking, of course, about the legendary Nedd Brockmann, a man who clearly takes the phrase 'cross country' far more literally than most.

In September 2022 Nedd laced up his runners and set out from Cottesloe Beach in Western Australia. He then ran 3800 kilometres across the continent over 46 days and 12 hours before finishing up in front of a cheering crowd on Bondi Beach. He averaged 80 kilometres per day. Nedd signed off his run with an Instagram post that summed up his superhuman effort:

> Australia: Ran it ✓
> 1.82 million dollars (so far): Raised it ✓
> Body: Cooked it ✓
> 11kgs: Lost it ✓
> Nation: Inspired it ✓

Mind: Lost it ✓

Sleep: Earned it ✓

Thank you all you bloody beautiful bastards xxx

Remember, GET COMFORTABLE BEING UNCOMFORTABLE.

The tagline that Nedd finished every post with – 'get comfortable being uncomfortable' – has become a much-hyped buzzphrase in recent years. Its origin is mysterious – many people credit it to the Navy SEALs – but today you'll hear it in CrossFit boxes and on motivational podcasts with increasing regularity.

The ubiquity of the line is fully justified, in my book.

YOU HAVE TO BE UNCOMFORTABLE IF YOU'RE SERIOUS ABOUT TRAINING TO ACHIEVE GENUINE RESULTS.

Weight training and cardio work heap stress on our bodies, and it's only through intense effort that we develop our strength, endurance and athletic performance. There's no getting around the fact that this process does entail some form of discomfort. You will sweat buckets. Your muscles will ache. You will find yourself gasping for breath. But it's only by building up tolerance to this stress that you can learn how to push beyond your limits and achieve physical and mental growth.

Admittedly, Nedd Brockman took the 'get comfortable being uncomfortable' memo more seriously than most on his run across Australia. Before he even started he was already experiencing mild shin pain and runner's knee in both knees. As his epic run unfolded, Nedd copped severe tenosynovitis in his shins and aggravated blisters. At one stage, his ankle became so swollen that he was left in crippling pain and unable to lift his foot or move his toes. But instead of abandoning his run, Nedd got a cortisone injection and ground out another 100-kilometre stretch.

The story of Nedd Brockman is a truly uplifting example of the value of a can-do mindset. Any one of the obstacles he faced during the race could've given him justifiable reason to quit. But he defiantly refused to cave in. Instead he tapped into the bigger goal of his charitable cause – his purpose. Nedd was running to raise money and awareness for the homeless and that helped to propel him onwards through the pain.

Embracing the phrase 'get comfortable being uncomfortable' doesn't mean you should do a Brockman and train through an injury. Nor does it mean you need to work out so hard that you puke or tear a bicep by taking on an impossible bench press. What it does mean is that, before your next serious workout, you should take a couple of minutes to mentally prepare. Brace yourself for the fact that at some point during your session the going will get tough. When your heart is hammering in your chest and your muscles are burning, quitting will feel like the easiest option. Serious exertion and stubborn effort will be required if you want to progress. Accept that reality before you start and prime your mind for the oncoming challenge.

For me, 'get comfortable being uncomfortable' simply means trying to strain through one final rep when it would be far easier to drop the dumbbells and take a breather. It's about trying to maintain your intensity as you attack that Tabata round of burpees right up until you hear the timer ring. It's about pushing hard in that final kilometre of your morning run when it would be easier to walk to the finish. Getting comfortable being uncomfortable means progressively turning up the difficulty rating of your workouts over time, instead of lapsing into a complacent plateau.

IT MEANS STRIVING TO INCH FORWARD EACH WEEK AND FINDING THE WILL TO PUSH HARDER.

Discomfort is an inevitable part of serious training. Whether you're straining to break a personal best on the squat rack or trying to run a half marathon in less than 90 minutes, at some stage you're going to come face to face with 'the suck'. Your muscles might start shaking or your limbs may be flooded with a tidal wave of lactic acid. At any rate, it isn't going to be pretty. In fact, the face of the suck is usually very ugly indeed. But rather than trying to avoid this scenario, remember that getting to know this character is what's going to help you to smash your goals. Making their acquaintance is a positive thing. It means you're on the right track to becoming stronger. Rather than recoil from the suck, you need to befriend them.

Someone I trained with who epitomised that mindset was UFC featherweight champ Alexander (Alex) Volkanovski. Obviously, he's a formidable athlete – at the time of writing he's number two in the UFC men's world pound-for-pound rankings – but what struck me in our sessions was his mental strength. As a trainer, I'm known for pushing people hard and wringing out every tremor of effort. But that still wasn't enough for Alex. I remember getting him to do a set of thrusters, an exercise in which you lift a barbell while explosively moving from a squat to an upright position. It's a full-body movement that requires a lot of energy and excellent technique. At the end of it, I gave him a 30-second countdown during which he had to bang out as many reps as he possibly could. At the end of that 30 seconds, most people collapse in a sweaty heap and rejoice that the ordeal is over. Not Alexander 'the Great' Volkanovski. When I called time, he ignored my call, gritted his teeth and kept going, somehow finding the reserves of spirit to crank out an extra 15 seconds. That was the moment I understood why Alex is the champion that he is.

THE MAGICAL POWER OF ROUTINES

Even if you're a hyper-disciplined person with a rock-solid mindset, your willpower has its limits. Perhaps the best way to picture your willpower is to imagine it like a muscle – think of it like your biceps, for example. If you work that muscle over and over again, hammering it with repeated sets, it's inevitably going to tire and become progressively weaker. It won't be able to perform effectively again until it recovers. It's the same deal with your willpower – it's a finite resource that you can't rely on forever. That's why you need good habits to prop you up when your motivation starts to waver. These positive routines can ultimately help automate your decision-making so you stay on the right track to achieve your goals with less effort. Sounds good, huh?

Positive habits have the power to help you take control of your health, your work and your family life (all the important stuff, in other words). But they're particularly handy when your life takes a darker turn. Let's say you lose your job or suffer a painful break-up. In those difficult moments when you're properly up against it, positive habits can hold things together when they could otherwise fall apart.

THE FLIPSIDE, OF COURSE, IS THAT BAD HABITS CAN DO THE OPPOSITE.

And when you're facing real adversity – the truly heavy shit – surrendering to bad habits can make it a lot tougher to bounce back.

Habits and routines can help you become more creative by freeing up valuable mental space. When your daily routine takes care of many of the humdrum decisions of daily life, it gives your brain more room to manoeuvre. Research shows that implementing regular work processes allows workers to spend less cognitive energy on recurring tasks, thereby allowing them to divert greater focus and energy to more involved tasks.[3] It's an idea endorsed by famed psychologist William James, who believed that only by regulating many aspects of daily life can we 'free our minds to advance to really interesting fields of action'. That's why it's a good idea to put your keys down in the exact same spot: so you don't have to waste precious time and energy hunting them down each time you want to leave the house.

The desire to conserve energy is the reason a lot of wildly successful people standardise their wardrobe by wearing the same clothes every single day. Steve Jobs stuck with a black turtleneck, blue jeans and New Balance sneakers. Mark Zuckerberg has a pile of identical grey t-shirts on repeat rotation. And while he was in office, Barack Obama consciously wore the same clothes day in, day out – limiting himself to a grey or blue suit. The reason, he explained in an interview with *Vanity Fair*, was to free up his mind for the important stuff. 'You need to focus your decision-making energy,' he said. 'You need to routinise yourself. You can't be going through the day distracted by trivia.'[4]

The good news is that it's a lot easier to form positive habits than you might think. You've actually formed a bunch of them already – it's just that they've become so instinctive that you now do them without a second thought. When you get into your car you automatically fasten your seat-belt. Every night before bed you religiously clean your teeth. Indeed, research shows that 43 per cent of what we do every day is performed out of habit.[5] The reason these positive habits have become second nature is down to one simple factor: you've repeated them day after day for as long as you can remember.

As any parent knows, we're almost hardwired to respond to routines. Babies and small children love the security of consistent patterns, whether that's time for a nap or something to eat. Routines offer a sense of reassurance and stability. Knowing they have that steadfast framework around them enables kids to play and learn without the unconscious anxiety that their basic needs will not be met.

So how do you form a new positive habit, whether it's hitting the gym on a regular basis or flossing your teeth every night?

As mentioned, repetition is the key. According to a study published in the *European Journal of Social Psychology*, the average amount of time needed for a set behaviour to become engrained is 66 days.[6] Not surprisingly, researchers also found that easier challenges tend to be more quickly integrated into your life than really complex ones.

Aside from the importance of repetition, following a few basic guidelines can help set you up for success.

GET SPECIFIC

Research shows that if the habit you're trying to develop is abstract or vague then it'll be a lot harder to stick to.[7] Your ultimate goal might be to 'get in shape' or 'lose weight', but those aspirations are too ambiguous and tricky to pin down. Instead you need to define the habit you're trying to stick to. So instead of saying 'I'm going to get fit', commit to a specific action. For example, you might say, 'I'm determined to work out for 45 minutes four times every week.'

BE REALISTIC

If your goal is too ambitious you're only increasing the likelihood that you'll ultimately fail. If it's achievable, you'll get confidence from your progress and hopefully set up a self-reinforcing positive loop. Rather than vowing to, say, run ten kilometres every day, whittle your goal down to something more manageable like running 30 kilometres over the course of the week. Once you've started to nail that task you can gradually crank things up.

FORM A PLAN

Researchers have found that you're far more likely to follow your routine if you've done the mental groundwork to determine when and where you'll do it and how you'll get there.[8] It's about thinking through the basic practicalities in advance, developing situational cues for your actions and working through the logistics. For example, instead of saying, 'I'm going to exercise three days a week', you might say, 'On Monday, Wednesday and Friday I'm going to stop at the gym for an hour on my way home from work.'

FIND A SWEETENER

It's human nature to respond to rewards, and research shows that you've got a much better chance of persisting with your regimen if it's fun.[9] It's worth building in an incentive, particularly in the early stages of developing a habit. For example, you might promise yourself an indulging massage if you hit your weekly exercise target; or, if you're trying to drink less, treat yourself to an ice-cream instead of a beer on an alcohol-free night. A joyless routine isn't just no fun, it's also far harder to stick to.

TRACK YOUR PROGRESS

If it's not measurable, it's not manageable. Self-tracking empowers you to know how you're really getting on. When you're trying to forge a habit, consistency is everything. Marking your wins on a calendar or app is a positive act of affirmation that can help you follow your plan with more conscious intent.

THE NUMBERS GAME

One client I trained who truly weaponised the power of self-tracking was the *Sunrise* weather presenter Sam 'Mac' McMillan. *Men's Health* had thrown down the challenge to see if he could go from 'dad bod to beach god'. It was my job to try to get Sam into cover-model shape. Unfortunately there were several complicating factors.

The first was that Sam had a properly crazy job. He was flying around for work all the time – at least two to three domestic flights a week, plus the odd international one. Being on the road so much meant it was really hard for him to settle into any sort of regular training schedule. The nature of his work meant that Sam would often find himself in random country towns on, say, a Monday night where the only available food options were the service station or the local pub. It was almost impossible to plan ahead.

As 'dad bod' suggests, the second obstacle was that just before I started training Sam he become a first-time father. Margot, his daughter, was only four months old when the transformation began, so Sam was understandably in that new-dad blur where his young family was very much his first priority. As a weather presenter, 3am wake-up calls were already the norm, but with a new baby in the house, his sleep was even more haywire than usual.

So we already had our work cut out, but then came the final curveball. Usually, to maximise the chance of getting impressive results, I like to spend 12 weeks on a client's transformation. But Sam had so much on his plate with family and work that he could only commit to eight weeks of training. Plus, due to the peripatetic nature of his schedule, we wouldn't be training one-to-one nearly as much as I would have liked.

A big part of the reason that Sam got the results he did and nailed his *Men's Health* cover was his willingness to commit to self-tracking. At the beginning of the challenge, he'd just got an Apple Watch that he was really into, so we used that to our advantage. The beauty of a smartwatch is that it holds you accountable. The numbers are there for you in black and white and you simply can't fudge them.

Due to the relative brevity of the challenge I posted a stiff target for Sam to aim for: I wanted him to try to complete 20,000 steps a day, plus 75 minutes of exercise. Every single day. To be honest, I didn't think that workload was realistic – but I wanted Sam to aim high, knowing that if he didn't reach that level he'd still be making progress if he got anywhere close. Luckily it turned out that Sam was a competitive bugger who'd represented Australia at international level in schoolboy soccer. He didn't want to let the Apple Watch get the better of him.

There'd be times, Sam told me, when he'd be in his hotel room after a flight and a long drive and it would be approaching 10pm, but he'd still be 4000 steps shy of his daily goal. So he did all sorts of crazy things to hit that 20,000-step tally – whether it was walking up and down his hotel balcony or running laps of the Bunnings car park. On *Sunrise*, he's on air every half hour from 5.40am, so between every segment he'd try to walk at least 1000 steps. By the time he got to midmorning, he was already at 10,000 steps, which was half of his daily allocation.

Sam's results demonstrated that some people can really benefit from self-tracking which, as I'll explain later in the book, can also be a great way to help you triumph over your vices by becoming more aware of your psychological triggers. Self-tracking also fortifies one of the other strong enablers for people who want to overhaul their health and fitness: accountability.

ACCOUNTABILITY IS EVERYTHING

It's difficult to overstate how significant accountability can be when you're embarking on a long-term health and fitness journey. Accountability is like having a personal trainer always looking over your shoulder and keeping you honest. It will register every workout with a nod of approval and wag its finger when you diverge from your good intentions. Personal accountability is the glue that fuses your commitment to your eventual results. It's the acceptance of responsibility and the refusal to make half-arsed excuses when you screw up.

There are different ways to make yourself accountable. One of the most effective is to spread the word about the goal you're working towards to as many people as you can.

IF YOU'RE TRYING TO ACHIEVE SOMETHING, DON'T KEEP IT TO YOURSELF.

One of my clients found great success with this by telling their followers on Instagram about their plans for the upcoming year. They posted a candid shot of themselves walking on the beach in athleisure gear and revealed that they were going to try to make some positive changes, including trying to cut back on sugar and junk food.

Doing something like that is a massive deal regardless of whether you have ten followers or a million. By making it public and keeping your following updated on your progress, you're declaring your intent to the world – which massively increases your personal accountability. If you fail to deliver, there'll be no place to hide. Your personal incentive will be greater than ever because no one wants to be seen as a public failure!

If you don't have social media, sharing your health and fitness goals with people you know is still a good idea. A study has shown that social support from friends and family is one of the single most effective ways to get people to stick to their exercise regimen.[10] Whether you're trying to lose ten kilograms or complete your first ironman, disclose that to your family, friends, colleagues or social media network. Sharing your goal with other people substantiates it. Instead of being a random thought in your head, suddenly it's official. It's harder for you to back out of it because, at some stage, someone will inevitably ask you how your challenge is going. You'll remember that when you are tempted to skip your training session or nix that plan for a run. Sharing your goals is an instant accountability generator that can help keep you on track.

If you're not a social media person there's a host of other ways you can crank up your personal accountability. Signing up to a competition like a Couch to 5K race or a Tough Mudder can be a good incentive – you won't want to waste the money spent on your entry fee. Or you could sign up to raise money for charity with an initiative such as Push for Better, which challenges you to complete a set number of push-ups during a specific time period.

Peer pressure is another great way to boost accountability. Consider tackling a joint fitness plan with a mate who you don't want to let down. Having a decent workout buddy can turbocharge your commitment. You're far less likely to miss a session if you know that, by doing so, you'll be piking on a friend. Plus it'll make your workout much more fun.

We all know that it's one thing to say you're going to stick to an exercise regimen, and another to follow through with it. Using these tricks to build a bulletproof sense of accountability can make all the difference to whether or not you ultimately go the distance.

MAKE YOUR COMEBACK BIGGER THAN YOUR SETBACK

The reason that accountability is so crucial is that you will face inevitable setbacks. Illness, injury and unexpected life events have zero respect for your desire to nail your goals. Everyone knows the path to success is rarely smooth.

WHEN CONFRONTED WITH A SETBACK YOU FACE A STARK CHOICE: YOU CAN EITHER USE IT AS AN EXCUSE TO PULL OUT, OR YOU CAN KNUCKLE DOWN AND FIGURE OUT A WAY TO KEEP MOVING FORWARD.

It's no surprise as to what I'd recommend you do.

One client I trained who exemplified the inner strength you need to handle multiple setbacks was the actor Hugh Sheridan, who I was training for another *Men's Health* transformation. I vividly remember our very first session together. I don't think Hugh particularly enjoyed it. Most people think of intense training as around 70 per cent of your maximum capacity. But when I'm training you, there's no mucking around or skipping reps. That proved a nasty shock to the system for Hugh. During that first session he was convinced he was going to puke. I don't mention this to embarrass Hugh – feeling nauseous is actually pretty common when you haven't trained for a while – but to stress how, after that initial experience, it would've been easy for him to start nervously looking for an escape route. And that was just the start of his trials.

Over the following months, Hugh was hit by a succession of problems that he could've easily used as excuses to quit. First up: I had to unexpectedly go to Los Angeles for work for three weeks, which interrupted the continuity of our training as we couldn't do one-to-one sessions. Armed with a detailed program, Hugh vowed to keep training on his own. Then COVID happened and all the gyms suddenly closed down. The logistical reality of training was now tougher than ever but, once again,

Hugh opted to stick with it. He bought some dumbbells and made a primitive DIY set-up on his deck to ensure he stayed on track.

From the beginning, the impetus for Hugh's transformation was the possibility of getting a *Men's Health* cover. But in the middle of his training, the magazine company changed hands and *Men's Health* stopped publishing abruptly (several months later it was acquired by another organisation and restarted). It was a brutal blow to Hugh's motivation. The original incentive for his transformation had suddenly been yanked away.

While all this was unfolding, Hugh had all sorts of craziness going on in his personal life, too. He'd moved back to Australia from the US after winning his dream role – he was to play the title character in a stage musical of *Hedwig and the Angry Inch*. This was where things became complicated. Hedwig is a character who is coerced into a sex-change operation as part of a convoluted plan to escape East Berlin. In Australia, some activists from the LGBTIQ+ community therefore considered Hedwig to be a transgender character and were angered that Hugh, rather than a transgender actor, had won the title role. Thousands of people signed a petition to have him removed from the role and, eventually, he did bow to the pressure to step down.[11] Adding a further dimension of personal complexity was that Hugh was also in the process of coming out as both bisexual and nonbinary – today he happily uses both he/him and they/them pronouns.

Looking back, what Hugh went though was a multicar pile-up of challenges. Facing those personal and professional issues, most people would have retreated to lick their wounds and recoiled from the additional stress of daily training. But Hugh kept going for two reasons. First, he realised how far he'd come already and didn't want his efforts to be in vain. Second, he realised that amid all this turmoil, the one thing he could control in his life was his training. And so he persevered, going on to achieve phenomenal results, dropping ten kilograms and getting down to eight per cent body fat. In spite of all the obstacles, Hugh kept moving forward, leapfrogging each setback in turn to get the job done.

KNOWLEDGE IS POWER

Every morning I used to crack 16 eggs in a row. I'd break one open, carefully bouncing the yolk back and forth between the two halves of the shell, letting the viscous egg white slop down into a tall glass underneath. It would take me about five minutes to repeat the process with each of the 16 eggs, until I had a glass full to the brim of raw egg whites. Faintly yellow in colour and with a texture not dissimilar to phlegm, it didn't look very appetising. Nevertheless. I'd hold my nose, glug it all down and desperately try not to gag.

I must have forced myself through that horrifying procedure every day for about six months when I was 18. Now I shudder to think about it. I must have knocked back about 1800 raw eggs during that time, sourcing them direct from a farm because buying them from the local supermarket would have left me bankrupt. The whole thing was totally insane and constituted a daily ordeal that I would dread. But I persisted because I was trying to bulk up. Back then, as a soccer-mad teenager, I weighed just under 70 kilograms. Today, 14 years later, I'm just under 100 kilograms.

That was my Rocky-style phase of egg-guzzling; you'll be glad to know that I never trained by pounding sides of raw beef in a meat locker. I mention this regrettable period not to promote this dubious practice, the mere thought of which now makes me retch. I bring it up to show how people can adopt really dumb ideas about the best ways to get stronger and fitter.

Accountability, mental grit, positive routines – developing all these will contribute to your success. But despite their undoubted importance, those attributes can still be fatally undermined if they're not backed by the right know-how. You can be full of energy, drive and commitment, only to start running in completely the wrong direction.

I read about that 16-eggs-a-day tactic on some dodgy bodybuilding website, which suggested quaffing raw eggs was the best way to get the protein fix needed to stack on serious muscle. Except that, as I gradually realised, it was, in fact, totally deranged.

I SEE THIS SORT OF THING HAPPENING ALL THE TIME.

A purported fitness influencer might post about a fad diet or weird routine that they claim has given them a seriously corrugated sixpack. Next thing, some impressionable gym-goer will start trying to implement the same program, but fail to get similar results. They get demoralised and start to think their training is futile. They might even be tempted to quit altogether.

The problem is that there's no one-size-fits-all dietary or training regimen that works for absolutely everyone. We all have different genes and rates of metabolism. We all have different injury histories and daily lifestyles, too. What works for me might not work so effectively for you. That's why mirroring another person's fitness habits – however impressive their results – often ends in tears. Or, in my case, revolting amounts of unnecessarily ingested egg whites.

In general, my advice is to be suspicious of any directives that promise to hold the secret knowledge to fast forward you towards your goal. There is no magic pill that'll help you lose your gut. There is no magical piece of gym equipment that you can buy from some late-night informercial that'll give you arms that look like an anaconda that just swallowed a pig. Even this book that you're currently holding in your hands doesn't have the single answer. What it does have is a broad series of principles and lessons that I hope will propel you on your way.

The reason I stopped necking that daily pint of egg whites is that I finally began to educate myself. I studied the latest research about protein synthesis. I discovered that eating raw eggs can lead to a biotin deficiency that can affect the metabolic process. I even found out that I'd been putting myself at risk of contracting salmonella. The more I learned, the more I realised that I could get the same dietary benefit from protein powders in a way that was far less stomach-churning.

All this begs an obvious question: there is now so much advice and information about nutrition – much of it contradictory – so how do you know what to trust? If, for example, you ask five nutritionists how many eggs you should eat each week, you're likely to get five different answers (although I'm fairly confident that none of them will endorse my 16-a-day habit). So how do you filter out the legitimate experts from those peddling broscience baloney? For me, I reckon you've got to give the advice-giver a critical once-over.

FIRST, DETERMINE THE BASIS OF THE PERSON'S CREDIBILITY.

If they're giving nutritional advice, for example, check whether or not they're a registered dietician. Scrutinise their track record, too. If they're offering fitness tips as a personal trainer, try to find out who they've trained in the past and how established they are in the industry. Doing a little bit of background digging is vital to assess whether the person's advice is really worth listening to.

SECOND, IT'S WORTH QUESTIONING WHETHER AN ULTERIOR MOTIVE COULD UNDERPIN THEIR POSITION.

If someone is constantly spruiking products, perhaps they're getting some form of kickback – whether that's financial or in some form of brand swag. All of this is a roundabout way of saying that you should always take influencers' suggestions with a degree of scepticism.

FINALLY, IT'S ALWAYS REASSURING IF A PERSON'S ADVICE IS BACKED BY OTHER PEOPLE OF AUTHORITY.

A bit of cross-referencing can not only deepen your insight of a topic, but allow you to see where opinions on the issue converge.

If you're putting in consistent effort, you deserve to get results. The amount of muddle-headed information out there is staggering. Don't fall victim to it. Educate yourself and learn to train smart.

PILLAR 2

EXERCISE

I was sitting down in the back room at my gym, Acero, with a new client. We were having an introductory powwow. The guy was carrying a fair bit of extra timber but his enthusiasm was palpable. He was itching to get started as soon as possible and commit to regular sessions. Before long, I drilled down to enquire about the physical results he wanted to aim for. 'Basically,' he replied, 'I want to get in shape for summer.' He went on to explain that he wanted to get bigger and stronger - adding size and definition to his arms, shoulders and chest. He also conceded: 'I want to lose my gut. Maybe even get my first-ever sixpack.'

Admittedly, these goals are hardly unusual. Most gym-going blokes want to supersize their arms and whittle down their waistline to reveal a set of rock-hard abs. The issue, which I had to gently break to my client, is that these two fitness goals are almost directly contradictory. In short, it's practically impossible to build muscle and lose fat at the same time.

Physiologically speaking, losing fat and building muscle work via oppositional forces. Building muscle is an anabolic process that requires a calorie surplus – you need to be consuming more calories than you burn. Conversely, losing fat is a catabolic process that depends on a calorie deficit. Trying to chase both at the same time will compromise your results in both areas.

It's for this reason that bodybuilders and fitness models typically approach their training in terms of specific cycles. They might, for example, commit to a muscle-building phase of six months, then change up their training and focus on a dedicated phase of fat loss. Unless you're a complete beginner – in which case you're almost guaranteed to see initial results with consistent training – I'd advocate a similar approach. If you're targeting a really serious physique, your best route to ripped is to focus on stacking on muscle first, before targeting excess fat by dialling down your body-fat percentage.

MUSCLE BUILDING 101

Before you embark on your muscle-building mission it's worth trying to understand the concept of hypertrophy. Essentially, this refers to the process that results in the boost in growth of your muscle cells. It's invariably triggered by resistance training as your muscles are forced to respond to the repeated stress. To accommodate being clobbered by the strain of all those reps and sets, your muscle fibres thicken. That's what strength training ultimately does to your body. You need to expose your muscles to this form of progressive overload if you want to stack on size. There are various ways of achieving this.

GO HEAVY

Sure, this isn't rocket science, but you're not going to build muscle and increase your strength with 2 kilogram dumbbells alone. Sometimes you have to train heavy. If you can lift heavier weights while maintaining good form and control, your muscles have to work really hard both concentrically and eccentrically. This workload damages the muscle fibres, which sounds bad but is actually a good thing. Your body repairs the damaged fibres by fusing them back together, thereby increasing the mass and size of your muscles.

Lifting heavy isn't something to attempt every time you hit the gym if you want to train consistently and avoid injury. But if you're serious about getting stronger, you do need to challenge your muscles.

GO SLOW

Slowing the motion of an exercise can increase your muscles' time under tension. The beauty of this strategy is that it removes the element of momentum, forcing your muscles to bear the full brunt – often at a painfully deliberate pace. I'll often prescribe a 4–2–2 cadence that involves lowering the weight for four seconds, holding it for two seconds, and then raising it for two seconds. If you can stick to that cadence while completing three or four sets, trust me: the burn will be insane. Slow and steady wins the (arms) race.

INCREASE THE MOTION

Another trick is to add extra quarter or even half reps to an exercise to increase the overall challenge. If you were doing a bicep curl, for example, this would involve adding an abbreviated quarter of the movement to each rep. That extra partial rep is just another way of increasing the amount of work that your biceps have to absorb and thereby further stimulates the release of muscle-growing hormones.

MIX IT UP

Muscles grow in response to stress. If you stick to the same moves at the same weights for too long, they'll get too comfortable. Instead you have to hit the same muscles in new ways by trying different weights, rep ranges and movements. If you always use a barbell for your strength work, for example, try to introduce more concentrated single-arm work. Alternatively, experiment with your foot positioning by standing on one leg rather than two, to destabilise your foundation and increase the overall challenge. Switching things up forces your muscles out of their comfort zone and should help prompt a physical response.

TRY GERMAN VOLUME TRAINING

This one isn't for newbies. German Volume Training (GVT) involves repeating ten sets of ten reps, concentrating on short recovery (60 seconds between sets) and a slow and controlled tempo. If you work at about 80 to 90 per cent of your maximum, this adds up to a super-taxing workout that will leave you sore the next day. But GVT does get results in terms of building strength in a certain movement or exercise. When you can complete all ten sets of ten reps, increase the weight by five per cent the next time around.

GET THE RIGHT FUEL

Exercise alone won't build serious brawn. Muscle building requires sufficient protein, as your body's calorific requirements rise in tandem with your physical efforts. If you're trying to gain muscle you can't afford to neglect this reality. The American College of Sports Medicine recommends that during hard training you should shoot for between 1.2 and 1.7 grams of protein per kilogram of body weight per day.[12] Ticking that box with regular food alone will prove a challenge, so top up using whey protein isolate to make up the shortfall.

EAT MORE, FULL STOP

There's a reason why bodybuilders eat five to eight times a day. To build muscle you need to chow down more calories. Maintaining a calorific surplus gives your muscles the raw materials required to repair tissue damage that's caused by heavy training.

TAKE CREATINE

Creatine is an amino acid derivative found naturally in muscle cells. It supports your muscles to rapidly create energy, an effect that's helpful during high-intensity or explosive exercise. As a result, it can help you to get stronger by enabling your muscles to handle more work in a single session. One study on weightlifters showed that creatine increased muscle fibre growth by two to three times more than training alone.[13] The best way to take it? Buy pure creatine powder and mix it with fruit juice – the sugar in the juice boosts your insulin levels, which helps your muscles absorb the creatine.

MEATHEAD MINDFULNESS

I wince when I see someone butchering their exercises with lousy form. Whether I witness someone bench pressing with flared elbows or attempting deadlifts with a hunched back, I often can't help myself and have to intervene. Lifting weights with poor technique is bad news, of course, because failing to engage the right muscles can easily lead to potential injury. If you don't do the exercise properly, you'll also never get the results your commitment deserves.

IN SHORT, YOU'LL BE SHORT-CHANGING YOUR TIME AND EFFORT.

That's why technique is absolutely crucial. Even with something as apparently simple as a bicep curl there's a lot going on. Contracting your arm to bring the dumbbell up and down is just one aspect. You also have to remember to keep your elbows locked in, to brace your knees to avoid harnessing extra momentum, to squeeze your glutes and to tense your abs as hard as you can.

It's worth using a personal trainer for at least some portion of your gym work so you can make sure you're nailing the details. Can't stretch to a personal trainer? Watch videos on YouTube or specialised fitness apps to ensure you're mindful of the fundamental principles when attempting a new move. Then attempt it yourself in front of a mirror and scrutinise the finer points of your form. If you're doing a complex lift, you might even get a mate to take a video so you can see yourself from every angle.

But visual feedback is only part of the overall picture. Another often overlooked detail is learning to tap into the mind–muscle connection. Arnold Schwarzenegger, a guy who knows a fair bit about maximising his gains, used to refer to this practice as 'meathead mindfulness'. As you execute any gym move, really focus on what your body is doing step by step. If you're doing a set of curls, concentrate on the position of your body to ensure your elbows are close to your torso and your upper arms are stationary. Exhale as you curl the weights up to shoulder level. While contracting your biceps, really zone in on the muscle you're flexing. Try to become aware of the physical sensation of the move, consciously noting the squeeze and savouring the tingle of pressure in the muscle at the peak of the motion. This targeted practice helps to enhance your muscle fibre activation, and research shows that it can lead to greater increases in muscle growth.[14]

Sometimes when life is hectic and there's a lot of mental noise it can be hard to muster the laser focus you need. To kill those distractions, try using a grounding technique to redirect your thoughts to the here and now – or, more pertinently, to the heavy metal object you're about to lift.

One of the most effective ways to tune your mind back into the present is using the 5–4–3–2–1 tactic. The idea is to pull your sensory awareness back to your immediate physical environment. To do this, stop for a second and mentally list five things that you can see right now, four things you can hear, three things you can touch, two things you can smell and one thing you can taste. Having recentred your consciousness to the present, try to maintain that sense of mindfulness as you do the next exercise.

Meathead mindfulness will improve your technique, protect you from injury and boost your results in the gym. It could also turn your workout into a form of mental release. Personally, what I love about exercising is that it's a chance to clear my mind and escape my problems or whatever stress is going on in my daily life. When I start training, I lose myself in the exercise and forget about everything else. The world melts away until it's just me and the piece of gym equipment that I'm using. That's what exercising does for me and why I love it so much.

WHEN YOU'RE IN THE GYM FOR 45 MINUTES YOU WANT TO GIVE EVERYTHING - NOT JUST PHYSICALLY, BUT MENTALLY.

EXERCISE FOR WEIGHT LOSS

Remember when I said that it's hard – if not impossible – to build muscle and lose weight at the same time? Well, I haven't changed my mind! If your primary goal is to lose weight, prioritise the exercises that will facilitate that quest. Those exercises will be different to those you'd recruit to build muscle.

NOT SURE WHETHER YOU SHOULD TARGET MUSCLE GAIN OR WEIGHT LOSS?

If you're counting down to a particular event – a beach holiday, say, or a wedding – and you have limited time to play with, weight loss can often make the biggest aesthetic difference to your physique. As the old saying goes, the easiest way to look like you've packed on five kilograms of muscle is to drop five kilograms of fat. Use the following principles to burn fat and hot wire your metabolism.

WALK MORE

People often ask me how I help my clients lose so much weight. The key to this transformation is very straightforward. One of the single best ways to lose unwanted body fat is by walking. It doesn't need to involve walking uphill, or carrying dumbbells, or that ridiculous-looking speed-walking you see in the Olympics. Simply walking for an hour a day will help you lose weight.

I appreciate that walking isn't the most earth-shattering tactic out there, nor will it be the only weapon you'll employ to lose your belly. But if you're trying to drop some kilos, you can't afford *not* to add walking into your weight-loss arsenal.

The beauty of walking is that you can do it every single day. It's not too hard or exhausting or unpalatable, so it's a practice you can add into your daily schedule without much difficulty. Catch the train to work? Jump off one stop earlier. Extend your dog's walk for an extra couple of kilometres (they'll love you for it). Make an evening stroll a relaxing part of your day by listening to a podcast or calling a mate while you pound the pavement.

The number of steps you do doesn't really matter, it's more about just trying to move more. For a basic yardstick, the standard goal of 10,000 steps a day is a good place to start. But if you can, start trying to nudge that up and aim for 12,000, 15,000 or even 20,000 like Sam Mac did. You don't have to lock in a set target, but having a daily goal can help make you more mindful of the tiny opportunities for extra movement you can weave into your day. A lot of my clients find that when they start monitoring their step count, they begin to take the stairs instead of the lift, walk to a colleague's desk on another floor rather than picking up the phone, or stroll around the park in their lunchbreak instead of dining al desko.

HIGHER REPS, MORE SETS

Years ago I worked at a gym where a competitive powerbuilder was training. While he was just an amateur, this guy was seriously strong: I'd regularly see him benching more than 160 kilograms. What fascinated me was his workload in the gym. He used to load up the bar with a scary number of plates – people in the gym would gawp – but when he started to lift, he'd always stick to low rep ranges, between one and five at the most. Then he'd take long rests – sometimes he'd wait ten minutes for his muscles to recover – before tackling the barbell once again. I could easily complete a 45-minute session with a client in the time it took for this guy to barely complete 15 reps.

The powerbuilder was training for hypertrophy by gradually increasing the weights, preparing his body to handle heavier loads from a neuromuscular perspective. It looked to be working, too. His priority was building monstrous strength, and he could indeed move a fearsome amount of iron. His physique was gigantic, too – he had the proportions of a wardrobe. He wasn't shredded by any means, and had a sizeable gut on him – but he was fine with that because he wasn't chasing a sixpack. He just wanted to get stronger.

I mention all this because if you're looking to lose weight you want to take the exact opposite approach to a power-builder. That means aiming for high reps and high set counts with minimal rest periods in between. Instead of three sets of ten to 12 reps with a 90-second breather in between, think five sets of 15 to 20 reps with 30 seconds' rest. With some clients, I even stop counting reps altogether and just get them to work for timed sets – about 60 to 90 seconds for each exercise. Using lighter weights allows you to increase the overall volume of your workload and the time your muscles are having to work. Keeping your heart rate high for this prolonged period will help you chisel away your excess fat.

CARDIO INTERVAL SETS

Try restructuring your cardio into fat-burning interval sets. This approach to cardio is essentially the opposite of going for a long, steady jog. It's hard yakka and it hurts, but it's very effective because it really gets your heart pumping. To do it, pick a cardio machine – let's say the rower – and set the timer for 60 seconds. During the next minute, go all out and try to cover as much distance as possible (you should definitely be panting by the end). Take a minute to get your breath back, then go again, repeating this process five times. On each cardio interval, track how far you go and try to keep the distance as high as possible. On the rower, aim to cover at least 300 metres on every attempt. For a running workout, do five sets of 60-second sprints at a fast speed. As I said, this isn't easy, but it's a workout that gobbles fat alive.

COMPOUND MOVES

Hoping to lose your love handles? Unfortunately it's almost impossible to target a particular area of fat on your body to spot reduce. If you're serious about losing weight, ditch the isolation exercises that pinpoint one muscle group at a time. Instead look to tackle big, compound exercises that work multiple muscle groups at once. Compound exercises rev up your heart rate higher than isolation exercises due to using large groups of muscles together. This makes them ideal for fat loss, so you want to do loads of them. Kettlebell swings, box jumps, burpees, thrusters, battling ropes and farmer's walks are just some of the exercises to involve if you're trying to get leaner and meaner.

IT'S NOT JUST ABOUT THE SCALES

If you know you're a bit heavier than you'd like to be and want to make changes I salute you and wish you the best of luck in your journey ahead. But I do have one important caveat: don't let the number on the scales rule your life.

As a personal trainer, I'm passionate about helping people exercise more, eat healthier and feel more confident and energised – but I've never advocated daily weigh-ins, and I'm even sceptical about weekly ones. That's because the number on the scale is liable to fluctuate by a considerable degree that has nothing to do with how much fat you've burned or how many calories you've eaten. There is a host of factors that can affect how much you weigh: hydration levels, medication, high-sodium foods, menstruation, sleep, alcohol, muscle mass and how recently you went to the toilet.

Your weight can vary by up to 2.5 kilograms during the space of a single day. That's a significant change in 24 hours and, if you're not aware of that possibility, it can become problematic. If the number has gone down, it can give you an unrealistic sense of your progress and risk inspiring complacency. But if you've been staying strong, eating clean and sweating bucketloads in the gym, seeing your weight randomly spike by a couple of kilos can be soul-destroying. Sadly, I've seen too many clients be demoralised by exactly that scenario. The next thing you know, they've suffered a nasty attack of the fuck-its, ditched the gym and settled down on the sofa with a packet of Tim-Tams to console themselves.

I am a big believer in tracking your progress, but there are more helpful indicators of where you are on your weight-loss voyage than the numbers on the scale. The first thing I always encourage a new client to do is to take selfies in their underwear in the mirror – from the front, side and back – and repeat the process at the beginning of every week. As any fitness model knows, lighting and the camera angle makes a colossal difference to how your body looks in any given photo. That's why you have to try to keep these measures consistent. Always take photos in the same mirror and ideally at the same time of day to try to negate variations in light. First thing in the morning is a good time to aim for.

At first these pictures are unlikely to make your heart sing with joy – but these private selfies will become the yardstick of your progress during the weeks and months ahead. Over time, you'll hopefully see your belly becoming flatter and the first inklings of definition around your shoulders, chest and arms. These pictures will ultimately tell a chronological story of your fitness odyssey – one that'll hopefully prove an inspiring tale with a feel-good ending.

Selfies are the simplest DIY measure, but other ways of tracking your weight-loss progress can include using a tape measure to take body measurements (waist, hips, thighs, chest and upper arms) or getting a monthly DEXA scan to get an accurate reading of your overall body-fat percentage. By all means check your weight on the scales, too – just don't live or die by the results.

PLAY THE LONG GAME

It's really important to keep your sense of perspective – particularly if you're on a long-term weight-loss journey. Nobody is perfect and you will screw up from time to time. Those blips are to be expected so don't let them knock you off course.

One of my clients brilliantly demonstrated this mindset when they were on holiday, staying at an all-inclusive resort where the food was so good, they felt like they had no self-control. As a result, they put on three kilograms.

For someone who's worked so hard to turn their health and fitness around, you might expect this news to have gone down really badly. But instead they made a joke about it on their socials. This relaxed approach was instructive. It showed how one little setback shouldn't make you lose sight of the bigger picture.

They showed a real sense of calm and practicality, reminding themselves that they could just get up tomorrow and go to the gym, and hydrate and eat healthy and love themself. After all, it hardly works to be hard on yourself.

In other words, you can always take the necessary corrective steps to recover if you slip up, but so often people take the all-or-nothing approach. They could be doing a sterling job with their diet and then succumb to a piece of birthday cake. Suddenly they start to catastrophise, and decide the damage is done and that they may as well make the most of it. They abandon their sensible eating plan and embark on a week-long binge-fest of junk food and booze. This logic makes zero sense. I mean, if you suffer a flat tyre, you don't slash the other three, do you?

What I loved about my client's approach was first of all that they were enjoying themselves on holiday, proving that they understand the true meaning of balance. Secondly, they've come to a place where they know that a number on the scales does not define who they are. Grasping those ideas is not only why they managed to lose a significant amount of weight with me, but also why they've subsequently continued to progress and become happier and more fulfilled than ever.

No one can be single-minded all the time, and holidays should be harnessed as an important opportunity to relax. When I go on vacation, I don't worry about training or what I'm eating. My holidays are for me to recharge mentally and physically. Enjoying them as much as I can enables me to return from them refreshed, re-energised and ready to get back to the gym with serious intent.

#45DAILY

So far in this section I've talked about exercise in fairly reductive terms. The reason I've focused on gaining muscle and losing weight is simply because those are the most common objectives most people who set foot in my gym have. Taking a more holistic view of exercise is a great way to improve your overall health. While I don't advocate daily gym sessions, nor do I suggest sitting on your bum on your days off. One of my most-used hashtags, #45daily, reflects that idea, and it doesn't take a genius to unpack its meaning. Simply try to incorporate 45 minutes of physical activity in some shape or form into every day.

There's a bunch of excellent reasons why taking on the #45daily mentality could help you.

I BELIEVE MANY OF US HAVE ADOPTED AN UNHELPFULLY NARROW VIEW OF WHAT EXERCISE CONSISTS OF.

Often we assume that physical activity only counts when it's based in the gym or a spin class or involves lacing up runners to pound the pavement. In other words it only counts if it's a tough, strenuous workout. Yes, that sort of exercise should be part of your overall regimen, but doing three or four gym sessions a week is only part of the equation.

In the world's longevity hotspots, such as Okinawa and Sardinia, structured exercise is rare. The people who live there aren't lyra-clad gym rats doing CrossFit sessions or HIIT workouts. They're simply living in environments that promote regular movement throughout the day. Their exercise is woven into the fabric of their lives – they walk, they bicycle, they garden. Rather than being stuck in a sedentary lifestyle, they're constantly on the move. That incidental physical activity adds up, too. You don't have to spend an hour in the gym every day to be healthy and lean.

Having a blinkered view of exercise is a self-sabotaging mindset because it will deprive you of a host of benefits. Just because you have a day when you can't make it into the gym doesn't mean that you can't still be taking positive actions towards your fitness or weight-loss goals. Cycling to work instead of driving, taking the stairs instead of the lift and having a walking meeting rather than sitting in an airless conference room are all useful ways to be more active. These forms of incidental exercise may not be too strenuous but they still contribute to your overall health.

SMALL HABITS CAN ALSO GIVE BIRTH TO LARGER KNOCK-ON EFFECTS.

I know one middle-aged guy who'd let himself go a bit and packed on the kilos. His New Year's resolution was to take 10,000 steps every day for the year. Truth be told, 10,000 steps is a modest daily goal that most able-bodied people can achieve if they put their mind to it. The effect on this client was profound. The first month, he walked his kids to school in the morning and went for a walk at lunch. After a while, he started going for a run first thing instead so he could complete his steps more efficiently. Soon he was smashing his 10,000-step target and decided to crank things up to the next level. First he signed up for a local parkrun and enjoyed it so much he decided to do a ten-kilometre race. Recently he did his first half marathon, and now he's training to take on the full 42.2 kilometre event. His experience demonstrates the value of setting micro-goals.

THE VALUE OF MICRO-GOALS

There are times when achieving a big health or fitness goal may feel like mission impossible. Will you ever be able to lose those ten kilograms or deadlift twice your own body weight? When your training quest feels unattainable it can become tempting to cut your losses and abandon ship. What you should actually do is embrace the power of micro-goals. As I always say to my clients: how do you eat an elephant? One mouthful at a time.

Looking at the big picture and strategically breaking it down into smaller pieces will always make things feel more manageable. You might have your overarching goal – for example, completing a marathon in under three-and-a-half hours. But that's not realistic from a standing start, so start by chunking it up. You might begin by targeting a ten-kilometre race after six weeks, or a half marathon after 12 weeks.

THE BEAUTY OF MICRO-GOALS IS THAT THEY GIVE YOU TASKS TO SUCCEED AT ALONG THE WAY.

You'll feel like you're making progress, giving you extra motivation.

If you like this idea, try splitting your overarching goal into monthly subgoals and weekly micro-goals. If you have a weight-loss goal in mind, focus on what you can achieve in the next seven days in terms of your habits rather than the number on the scale. You might, for example, aim to exercise five times in the next week, have four alcohol-free nights and pack healthy lunches for work rather than resorting to the greasy cafeteria.

Something I remember from my soccer days is just how powerful a force momentum can prove. If you play for a team that starts winning, the collective levels of confidence and self-belief rise. Your once-jittery defence can suddenly gain composure; your striker can start taking more shots and scoring more goals. The opposite also applies: if your team is stuck in a losing streak copping defeats game after game, it can become harder to break out of the rut.

Setting a series of achievable micro-goals can help you to harness the power of positive momentum. You can then draw encouragement from that and surf the wave of success to your ultimate goal. Bite by bite you'll polish off that elephant in no time.

Enough about goals, Jono, you might be thinking. *I want some tools and tips I can use to improve my actual workout!*

Well, fair enough. Let's get into the nitty-gritty, and talk about how you can improve your workout with a bit of imagination and careful planning.

USING IMAGERY TO UNLOCK YOUR NEXT PERSONAL BEST

Sports psychology and its principles are fast becoming a popular tool among athletes striving for peak performance. More and more often we hear about athletes at the top of their game utilising psychological techniques to perform at their best. Imagery (also known as visualisation) is a technique whereby a skill or the performance of a task is visualised in one's mind. So how can we apply it in our day-to-day workouts?

IMAGERY AND COGNITIVE REHEARSAL

In the 200-metre butterfly event at the 2016 Olympics, Michael Phelps was the hot favourite to claim yet another gold medal. But as soon as Phelps dived in, his goggles broke and filled with water.

Phelps went on to win the race while being essentially blinded the whole time. How did he do it? Well, Phelps credited his mental preparation, including his visualisation process, for being able to perform as well as he did. He said that he had already swum that race hundreds of times in his head and had visualised what he wanted it to be – but more importantly what it could be, taking all possible scenarios into consideration.

Imagery has been consistently reported to enhance physical performance in a variety of sports. More specifically to the training world, imagery has been linked with performance increases in motor, power and strength-related tasks through improved technique and execution. Additionally, imagery can have a positive effect on psychological states and ultimately enhance self-confidence and motivation while limiting anxiety. Pretty neat, huh?

It's no surprise that it has become a popular mental skill among competitive athletes.

So, how can simply imagining a skill help to improve it? The psychoneuromuscular theory explains that when a task is visualised, the same muscles that are used in the actual task are innervated. With repeated practise, the motor performance of these skills can improve.

Imagery can be used specifically to:

- Practise a skill that has yet to be perfected
- Maintain and refine existing skills when physical practice is not possible
- To get focused immediately prior to during competition
- Increase self-efficacy
- Prepare for competition
- Improve psychological skills

THE PETTLEP MODEL OF IMAGERY

For imagery to be effective, the visualisation itself needs to be as vivid as possible. The PETTLEP Model of Imagery, developed by Holmes and Collins in 2001, provides a framework to create as vivid an image as possible.

Summary of the PETTLEP Model of Imagery

Physical

Physical state of the imager should mimic the arousal level and body position of the behaviour during performance. Essentially, even if you don't have weights with you at home, you can practice technique by literally going through the motions.

Environment

Use the environment in which athletes perform to engage in imagery. If you're practising chest presses on your couch, imagine being at your gym or wherever you exercise. Try to bring in as many details as possible.

Task

Consider the nature of the task being imagined and its interaction with the skill level and ability (i.e. technique, range of motion, and weight). Home in on the thing you're trying to improve: the angle of your limbs, for example.

Timing

Imagine the event or task in real-time to ensure it mimics the actual performance. Don't just skip through!

Learning

Consider the trajectory of learning and skill development to refine images accordingly. What's your goal?

Emotion

Use emotion when creating and engaging in imagery to stimulate what is felt when performing the behaviour. How do you feel about what you're working towards? Use it for fuel!

Perspective

Imagine the event or situation through the perspective of one's own eyes. Visualise it in the first person, not as an out-of-body experience.

Using Imagery to Enhance Lifting Performance

So, it's clear that we can use this mental skill to enhance our lifting. Here's how you might go about visually preparing to squat a new personal best, for example:

FROM YOUR OWN EYES, IT'S IMPORTANT TO VISUALISE WHAT WILL BE HAPPENING BEFORE EVEN APPROACHING THE BAR.

You might start by going through your pre-lift routine, creating the exact feelings and emotions that you anticipate. Will you be standing, walking around, or sitting down calmly? Where possible, include as much detail about the environment as you can. Next, you may increase your arousal in anticipation for the lift, perhaps you visualise standing up and approaching the bar. Are you listening to music first? Include it. As you approach the bar, visualise the plates you'll see and as you grab the bar, imagine what the knurling feels like in your hands. Think of the feeling of having the bar on your back as you un-rack it, and your confidence as you do so. Hear the sound of the bar popping out of the rack as you stand and the feeling of stepping back with the bar. As you start the squat, imagine it in real-time, descend as slowly as you usually would and come up confidently out of the squat.

Visualisation can be practised before, during and after the exercise. For preparation, you may like to include it some weeks away from training right up until before the task. Do it after, too – rerun the things that went right or wrong!

LIMITING FACTORS AND HYPERTROPHY

Visualisation isn't the only tool in your workout box. Exercise selection to maximise hypertrophy is one of the training variables that I consider when designing a hypertrophy program for my clients, and it can make a huge difference. There are a few factors we need to take into account. One is the limiting factor of that exercise.

First, let's just refresh on how we maximise hypertrophy in training. The goal in training is to provide a stimulus of sufficient magnitude and duration to elicit a hypertrophic response. Basically, we need to perform our exercises with enough load and to a sufficient relative intensity, which means taking our working sets 3–0 reps from failure.

So we've established that to grow a muscle we must stimulate that muscle. So which exercises achieve this best? Well, what you need to know is that muscles don't recognise exercises. Your quads don't know if they are doing a leg extension or leg press. Both will stimulate the quads, so both will cause growth.

THIS MEANS AT ITS MOST BASIC LEVEL, YOU CAN PICK ANY EXERCISE YOU LIKE, AS LONG AS IT TARGETS THE DESIRED MUSCLE GROUP AND YOU WORK HARD ENOUGH WITHIN THE SET.

A limiting factor is essentially the component of a system that will be the first to fail. As it relates to hypertrophy, we want to make sure that the limiting factor of an exercise is the target muscle group.

I'll give you a (somewhat contentious) example. Front squats are often programmed with the goal to increase quad stimulation, as opposed to a high bar or low bar back squat. It's true that quad emphasis is increased in a front squat in comparison to its counterparts due to the front rack position of the bar, allowing the lifter to keep a more upright torso position and increase knee flexion. This means the quads are being moved through a greater range of motion. This sounds great, but I'd argue that in a majority of cases the limiting factor for people doing front squats is thoracic strength (their ability to hold the bar in the front rack position). If you have to drop the bar before your quads have been stimulated, then is this an effective exercise to stimulate growth? Probably not. A better use of the front squat would be if you find that your torso collapses coming out of the hold, and you want to increase your strength in this position. In this case, you'd probably program in another secondary squat session and it wouldn't be the primary exercise for your quads.

Other common examples include:

- **UNSTABLE SURFACES:** Completing exercises on unstable surfaces will more than likely reduce the amount of load you use or reps you can complete. Are you using the exercise to stimulate your target muscle or train your balance?
- **GRIP STRENGTH:** Often in the gym you'll see people continually dropping weights or ending sets early as their grip strength is failing. They'll then say things like 'It's all good, my grip strength

> just needs to catch up'. Sadly, it rarely does – and while it's a good idea not to simply use wraps and chalk for every exercise you do, your deadlifts are not going anywhere fast if all you care about is grip strength. If grip strength is a priority for you, then there are a number of different and specific exercises for this that don't interfere with the development of other body parts.

If maximising hypertrophy is the goal, then the target muscle must be the limiting factor for that exercise. If this isn't happening, then it's likely that the target muscle group isn't being effectively stimulated. The good thing about this concept is that it's very straightforward to tell whether you're targeting the appropriate muscle – you'll feel it!

The other factor that works in our favour is that hypertrophy can be achieved through any exercise.

THIS MEANS THAT THROUGH EXPERIMENTATION YOU CAN FIND EXERCISES THAT BEST SUIT YOU.

TEMPO & TIME UNDER TENSION

Two common terms we hear in gyms are tempo and time under tension (TUT). The reason why I think this is important is because both tempo and TUT are misinterpreted and therefore often misapplied. Firstly, tempo and TUT are not the same. Secondly, they are not a 'type' of training. You don't 'do' a TUT program! Every time you train, you are spending TUT. Tempo is a training variable that we manipulate within training. The most common way that these two concepts are misunderstood is when someone believes that significantly slowing down their repetition speed (tempo) increases the TUT they achieve in an exercise, and is consequently superior for growth.

I'm sure you've seen the bros doing 5 second eccentrics on every set of every exercise because it 'increases their TUT'. (I've been one of them.) But this isn't necessarily the case.

TIME UNDER TENSION

First things first, muscle hypertrophy is achieved through applying tension of an appropriate magnitude and duration to the target muscle. The magnitude will dictate the adaption that occursinsert: i.e. higher magnitudes (loads) will elicit more strength and lower magnitudes will bias hypertrophy. The duration refers to the dose or how much of that tension or stimulus is being applied.

FROM A RESISTANCE TRAINING PERSPECTIVE, THE MORE WE CAN DO AND RECOVER FROM, THE BETTER OUR PROGRESS IS LIKELY GOING TO BE.

So yes, duration of tension and therefore TUT is important within training ... but is this achieved by significantly slowing down your reps? Let's compare two different sets of bicep curls:

- Subject 1 completes their bicep curls at a regular cadence. They focus on squeezing the muscle hard at the end concentric and then lower the weight at a speed that is conducive of them being in control i.e. not letting it drop.

- Subject 2 starts the same but now takes five seconds to lower the weight.

Subject 2 will be spending a lot longer performing each rep, but why does Subject 2 not necessarily have a better stimulus? The main factor is because that Subject 1 will likely get a lot more reps. So while Subject 2 may have more TUT per rep, Subject 1 will complete more of them. So, it could be argued that the amount of TUT for both subjects is similar.

What's important is achieving enough stimulus per set to elicit a hypertrophic response and we do this by taking each set close to failure (with 0–3 reps in reserve (RIR)). If you do a set of eight curls with a five-second eccentric vs a set of 15 curls at normal cadence, then as long as they reach that point of close to failure then you're on the right track.

Slowing down the speed at which you perform an exercise will probably still be effective for muscle hypertrophy, but there can be a catch. It's likely that using slow eccentric training as a means of increasing TUT can be taken to a point where it becomes detrimental to one's progress.

Firstly, let's consider session volume. As a general rule, when hypertrophy is the goal we want to spend most of our time working in rep ranges of 6–20. If you find that because you're significantly slowing down the speed of the movement to increase TUT, but now 50 per cent of the sets you do in your workout are in the 3–5 rep range, then you are cutting your training volume significantly and likely too much to optimise hypertrophy. Generally, if we're in the 3–5 rep range, the loads we are using will push some gains in strength. But we don't even get that anymore because the loads we have used for slowed eccentrics are too low.

Second is recovery. It's well documented you can cause increased muscle disruption or damage from doing heavy eccentric work in your training.

WHILE THIS SOUNDS APPEALING FOR GROWTH, YOU CAN ALWAYS HAVE TOO MUCH OF A GOOD THING.

If you are constantly sore and under recovered because all you do in training is extremely slow eccentrics, then your ability to grow will likely be hindered because you aren't letting your body recover. If you can't recover from training, then your training volume will drop and you'll also be more likely to get injured. No thank you!

TEMPO

Tempo refers to the actual speed we perform each part of an exercise. Exercises we perform are commonly categorised as concentric or eccentric, and then further into concentric, end concentric, eccentric, end eccentric. If you are unsure what this means, concentric is the shortening of a muscle and eccentric the lengthening of a muscle. When someone says they are doing 'tempo' training in order to achieve a better stimulus (which isn't a thing, remember?), they are essentially manipulating the speed of these phases in the movement. As we have already discussed, slowing down the tempo does not necessarily equate to increased stimulus just because you are performing the movement slower – and can even be detrimental to growth if taken to the extreme.

So what is the best application of tempo and how may this lead to a more stimulative exercise or session? Think about whenever you have learned a new skill! You don't start by trying to perform it at full speed. To fully piece it together you usually have to slow the movement down, slow parts of the movement down or even break movement down into segments. Well the same applies for exercises in the gym. If someone has technical issues with their squat that as a coach we want to address, it's likely a good idea to give them a slowed tempo. In this example a three-second eccentric with a two-second pause would help them better think and coordinate the movement, rather than have them dive bomb into the hold and come straight back up. Slow down the descent and take time to think about bracing, where your knees should be tracking, feeling the bar on your back. Just like with any other skill, the more you practice the more automatic it comes.

If you use tempo as a means to improve technique, this is actually a time where coincidentally you will achieve a greater TUT on the target muscle as opposed to a faster cadence for the same exercise. For example, let's say for Romanian deadlifts the only thing you feel is your lower back. It turns out that when looking at your technique, the movement is not actually coming from you hinging at the hips at all but rather your spine that is flexing to lower the weight. Now that you've seen this, you slow the eccentric part of the movement down and focus on pushing your hips back the whole time with a neutral spine – and now your hamstrings and glutes are smoked! You've taken the same exercise from poor technique and working your spinal erectors to good technique and working your glutes and hamstrings. That's how you would increase TUT for the target muscle using a tempo.

As you become more and more proficient at that exercise you will likely remove that slower tempo and find a speed that simply allows for control of the movement with heavier loads.

KEY TAKEAWAYS

- Tempo and TUT are not forms or styles of training. Tempo is a training variable.
- Slowing reps down to increase TUT does not necessarily equate to a greater stimulus as more reps can be completed at a normal rep cadence.
- Excessively slowing down your exercises to increase TUT may actually have detrimental effects on hypertrophy if volume demands are not met. It may also increase your likelihood of injury from poor recovery.
- The main use of tempo should be to help improve technique.

- Improved technique using a tempo may actually increase TUT on the target muscle as you are correctly training that muscle.

PEBBLES VS STONES

What do we get if we throw pebbles into a lake? Small ripples that quickly subside. There is little disturbance or change to the large expanse of water. How about a heavier stone? Well, there's a splash! Water flies everywhere and the disruption it causes to the once still lake is pretty significant. But what does this have to do with your fitness journey?

I strongly believe that one of the biggest reasons that people struggle to achieve any health and fitness goal is because they put too much effort (or none at al) into the pebbles. What are some examples of pebbles in health and fitness?

- Fat-burning supplements (most supplements, for that matter).
- Whether you do your cardio before or after you have eaten.
- When you eat carbs and what type of carbs you eat.

- Consuming protein within ten minutes of finishing a workout.

To explain why these are pebbles, I need to tell you what some of the stones are:

- Energy balance
- Protein intake
- Adherence to your fitness regime
- A healthy mindset around training, nutrition and the body
- Appropriate resistance training that:
  - Is specific
  - Is performed with correct technique
  - Follows a progressive overload

For now, let's keep this discussion to physique-based goals. What I'm getting at is that if you put more time into the stones, you will elicit a far greater result in comparison to putting your effort into the pebbles. If you're trying to drop body fat but don't have your energy balance in check, then no fat burner in the world is going to help you.

When you look at it, it makes perfect sense. Focus on the things that you have to do in order to achieve your physique goal. Using fat loss as an example again, for the goal of fat loss, you have to be in an energy deficit. You don't have to use a fat burner or do your cardio before eating to lose fat. So why are these the things that people put most of their thought and effort into?

WELL, IT DOESN'T TAKE MUCH EFFORT TO PICK UP A PEBBLE AND THROW IT.

A stone on the other hand is heavier. You'll have to squat down, use two hands and then give it a huge full-body swing just to get it over the water's edge. It's tough to begin with, but once you get over that initial barrier, the effect is huge. It's easy to buy a fat burner and chug a scoop every morning hoping you'll have abs by the end of the day. It takes more effort to sit down with a coach to get real and honest about your current nutrition and what needs to be done for you to make long-lasting change. I believe that we all know what has to be done, but facing it is the issue – especially when we are constantly promised easier and quicker solutions. Believe me, if you told me that I could keep my shitty diet and all I had to do to

get lean was do cardio for an hour before I eat, I'd be all over it.

This being said, the pebbles have their place ... but only when you have thrown all the bigger stones. They have the potential to give you that extra boost in your training and nutrition, but I can't stress enough how useless they are without the key foundations in place.

IN SUMMARY, IF YOU WANT TO CREATE LONG-LASTING CHANGE, THEN YOU HAVE TO DO THINGS THAT MAKE WAVES.

PILLAR 3

NUTRITION

What's the secret to everlasting happiness? It's a big question to which many of the world's brightest minds have offered their wisdom. Some believe happiness lies in the quality of your relationships; others say it requires a certain level of financial security; some believe it's about cultivating a highly developed sense of gratitude. Unless I've missed something, none of the great philosophers have ever suggested happiness requires subsisting on an extreme diet or trying to get to seven per cent body fat.

I suspect there's a good reason for that, too. There have been times, particularly early on in my career, when I've dabbled with a very strict diet for a while (I mentioned eating 16 eggs a day for six months). But it's never been an enjoyable journey, so I've inevitably ditched it before long. Yes, if you want a sixpack you can grate cheese on, you do need to get your body-fat percentage way down into single figures. But making the necessary sacrifices to get you there is unlikely to make you happy. Instead, it's likely your relationship with food will be riddled with longing, anxiety and guilt. This is why heavily restricted diets rarely work out for anyone long-term and invariably turn into a binge-and-purge cycle as your weight yo-yos up and down. The single biggest mistake I see clients making with their nutrition is putting too much pressure on themselves.

Most people will soon feel utterly overwhelmed if they're weighing all their meals and painstakingly counting every calorie. Unless you're a fitness model, a professional athlete or some sort of number-crunching control freak with masochistic tendencies, that strategy will simply be too hard and is more likely to derail your good intentions.

What bothers me about so much nutritional chit-chat in the health and fitness arena is that it often tends to push for extreme restriction. Whether it's the paleo diet (no grains, legumes or dairy), the keto diet (no carbs) or trying to remove some other culprit be it gluten, lactose, sugar or processed foods, I believe the risks often outweigh the rewards – unless, of course, you're cutting these things out on the basis of medical advice. Instead, I prefer to promote broad principles that are easy to stick with and that actually work. Life is too short to live on protein shakes and joyless meals.

EAT TO BE SATISFIED, NOT FULL

I've never been to Okinawa in Japan, but I feel like there's a lot I could learn there. The Okinawans have one of the lowest rates of illness from heart disease, cancer and stroke in the world, as well as enjoying one of the highest life expectancies. I'm also fascinated by a concept that originated there – *hara hachi bu* (eat until you're 80 per cent full) – that nails how I believe we should approach our meals.

Most people in the West have an increasingly twisted idea of portion control. We think we need to eat far more than we actually do. For many of us, this belief has its roots in our childhood. Coming from Colombia, a poor country where a lot of people struggle to feed their families, my mother always impressed on me how important it was to

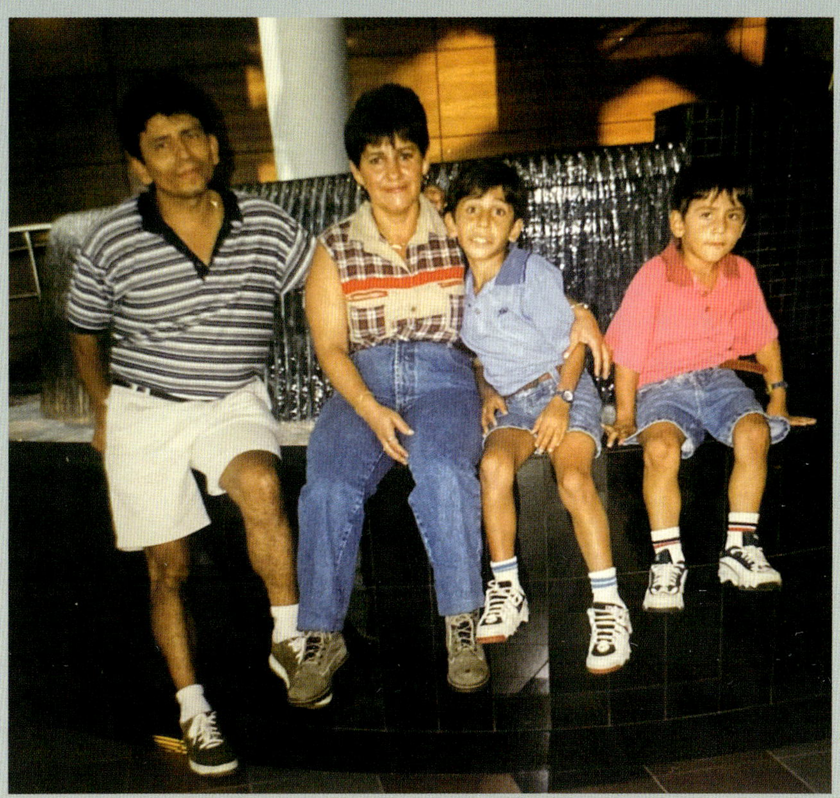

My amazing family, without whom I never could have got this far. I'm the kid on the right in each photo, but you can see my brother and I are pretty clearly related. My family have always been so supportive of my goals – it's hard to believe how much has changed since then!

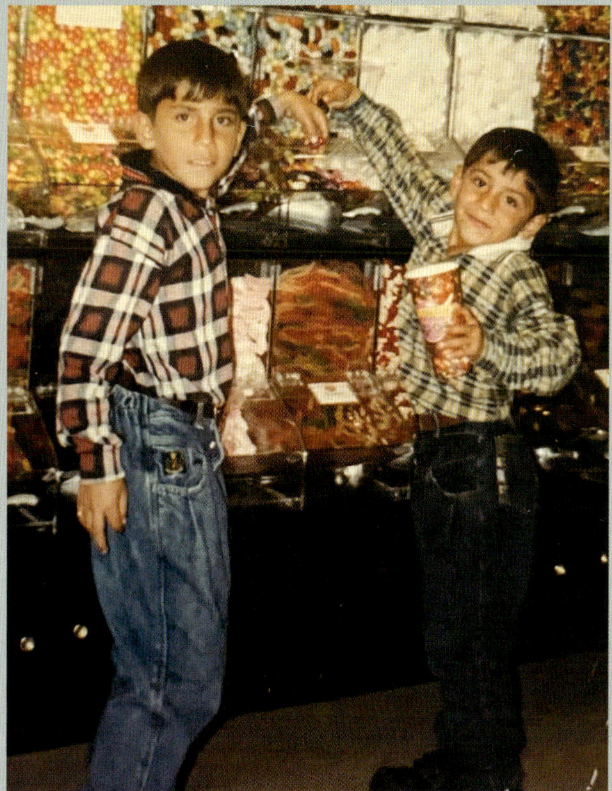

PEPSI

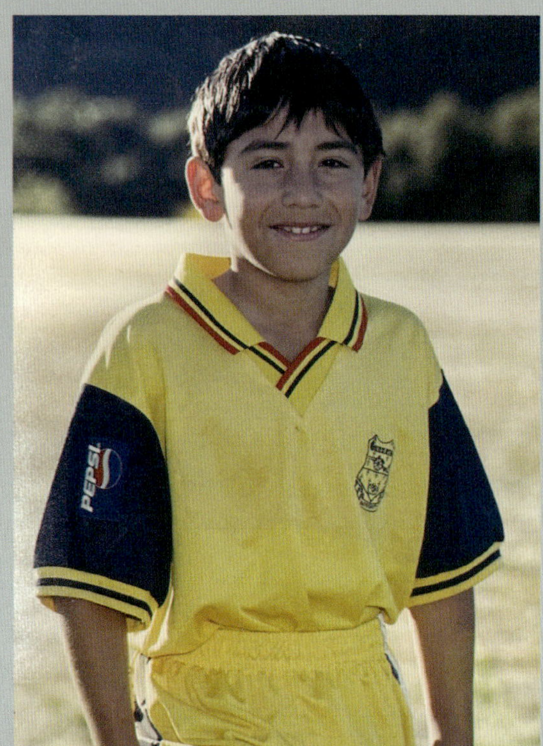

Though I wasn't to fulfil my childhood dream of becoming a professional soccer player, it was all part of the journey (and definitely helped with building a foundational level of fitness!).

U12's Bankstown City Cubs 2003
Front Row: N.Kapsis, D.Ralevski, J.Kapsis, N.Fernandez, A.Rasimoglou, J.Soilemezidis, T.Nolevski
ack Row: B.Stankovski, T.Taylor, E.Schlack, J.Smith, T.Murtanovski, B.Bogoevski, S.Calic, J.Castano
Coach: Richard Machado
Manager: Anna Smith

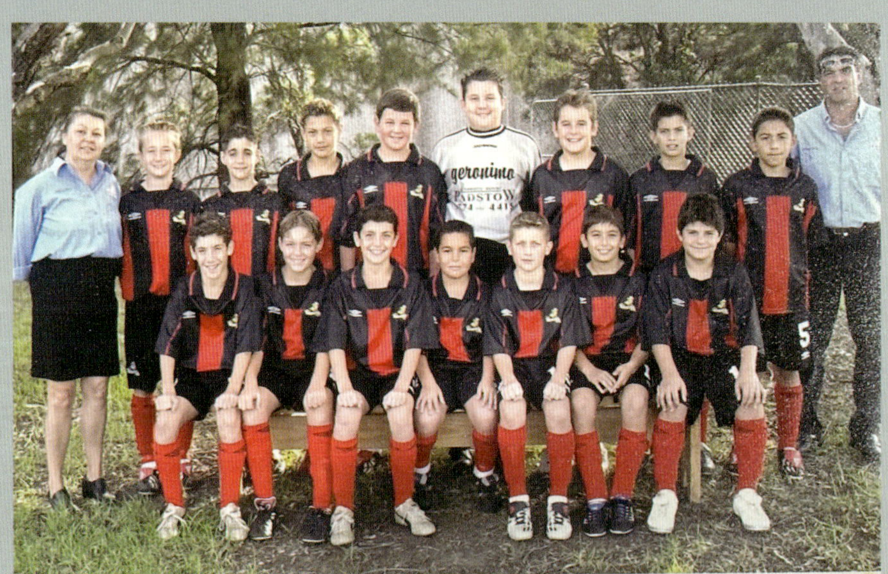

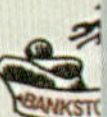

Joel Creasey's before-and-after. What a legend! (And, of course, a brilliant comedian.) It was amazing to see his progress first-hand. Joel worked out two hours a day, even flying between Sydney and Melbourne several times a week for fitness classes. He ended up shedding 12kg of fat and putting on 4kg of muscle. (*Men's Health*)

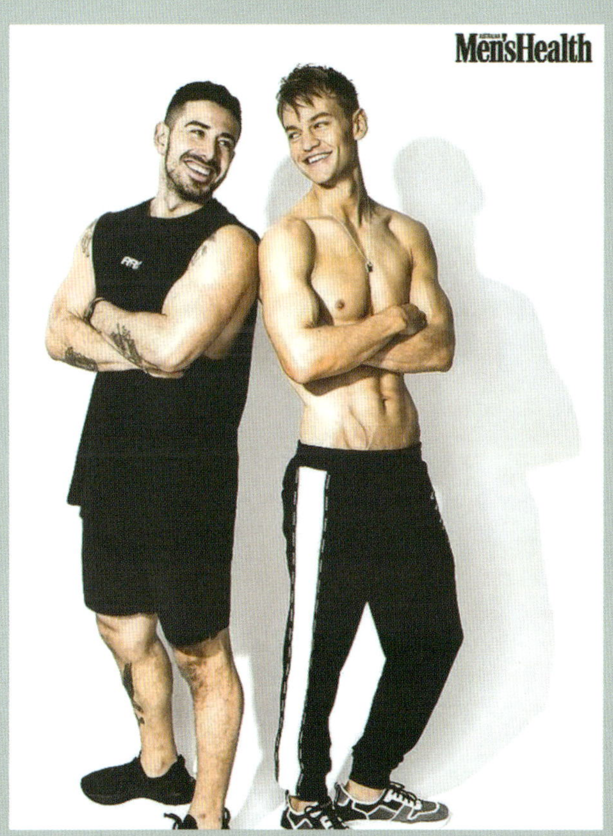

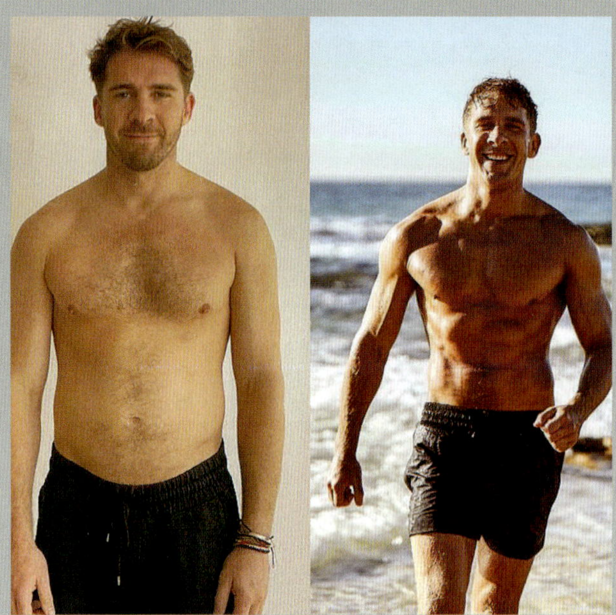

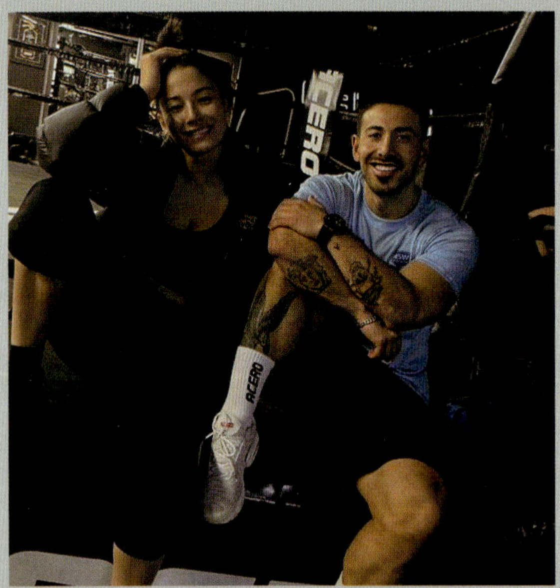

Above: Hugh Sheridan, known for *Packed to the Rafters*, was fantastic to work with, and his before-and-after is a testament to his dedication. He made the big holistic changes that really carry you through a fitness regime, and all that hard work paid off, as you can see!

Left: Jessica Gomes, Aussie supermodel, is one of our regular Acero visitors.

Right: My lowest moment, and highest weight.
Below: My before-and-after.

This was the roughest patch of my life, but in retrospect it also was the best moment for me to reconnect with my values and find myself.

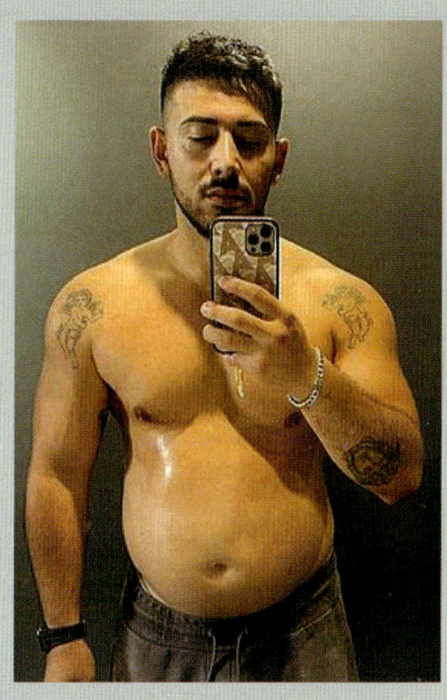

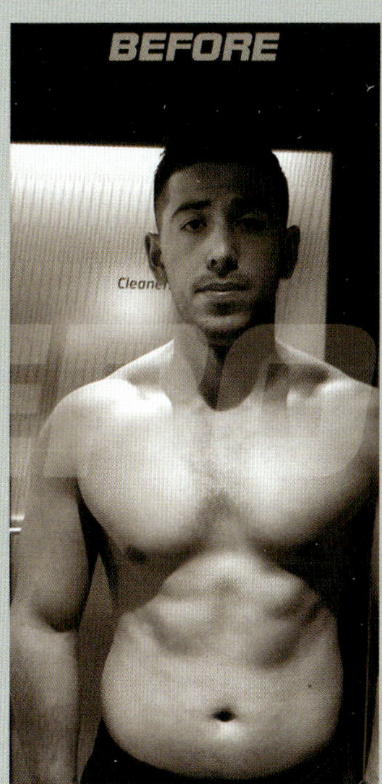

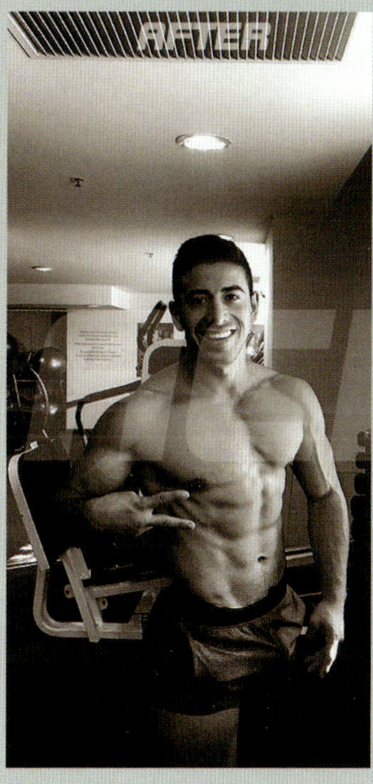

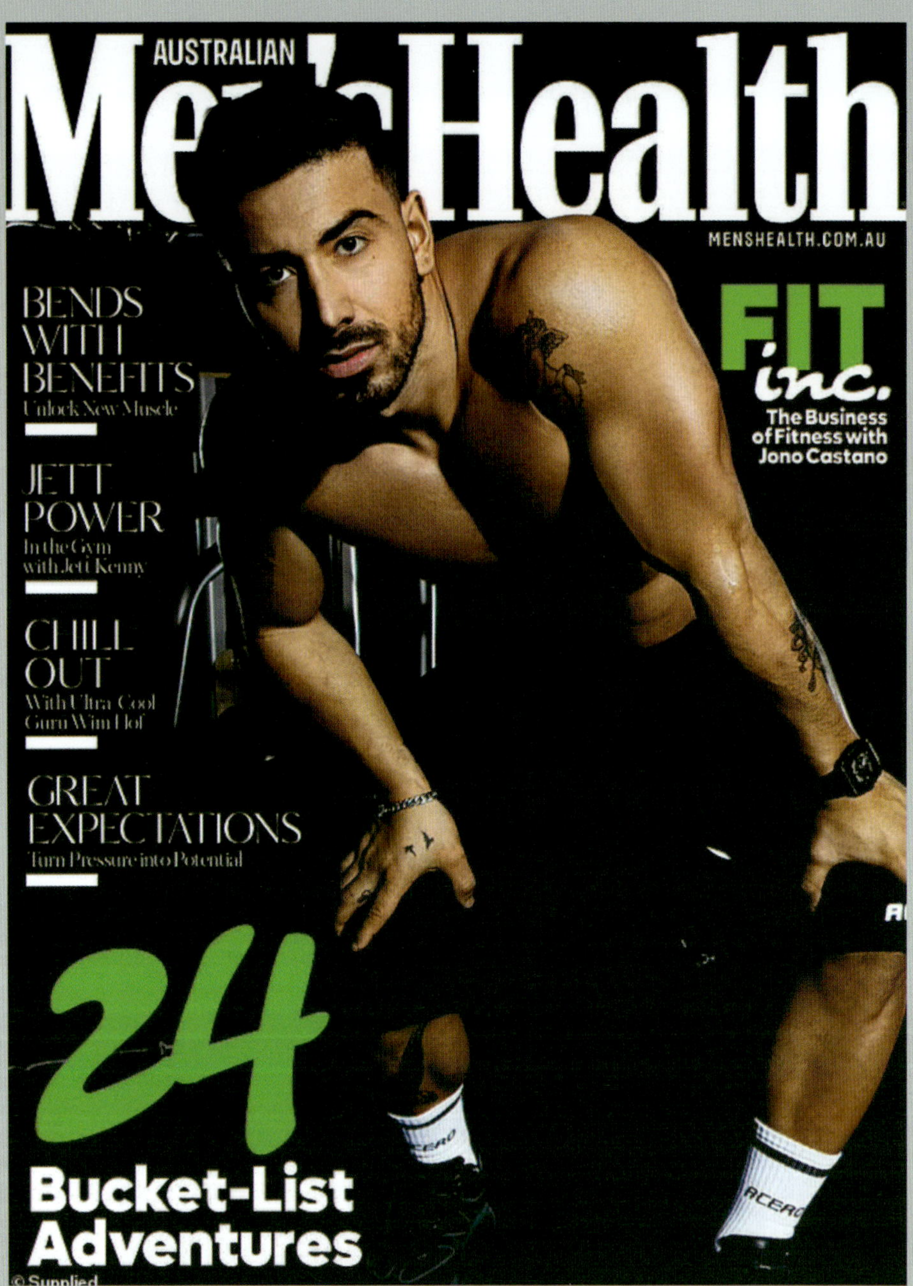

All my hard work had paid off by the time I did the shoot for this cover. Working with *Men's Health* was a blast – and provided some welcome pressure to get myself back in shape. (*Men's Health*)

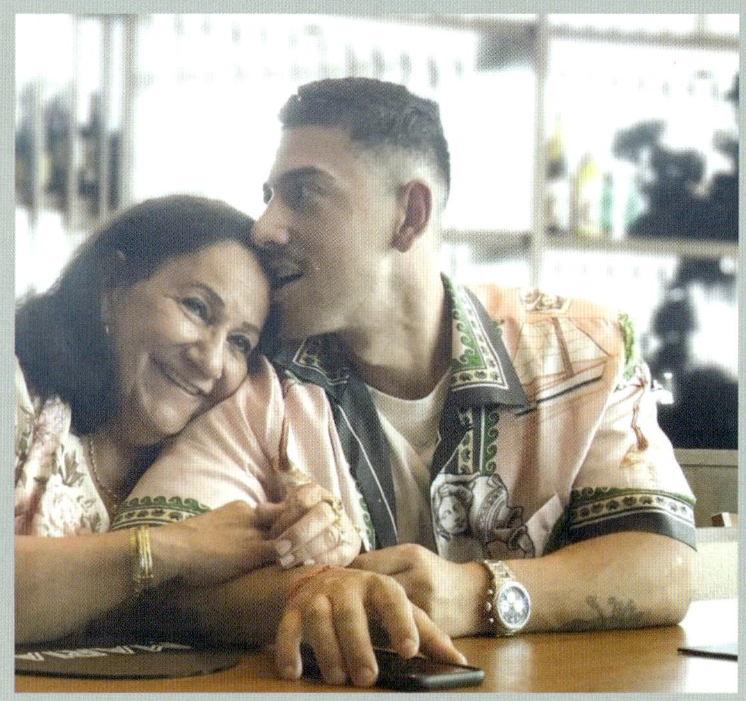

What would I do without my family's support? It's all thanks to them.

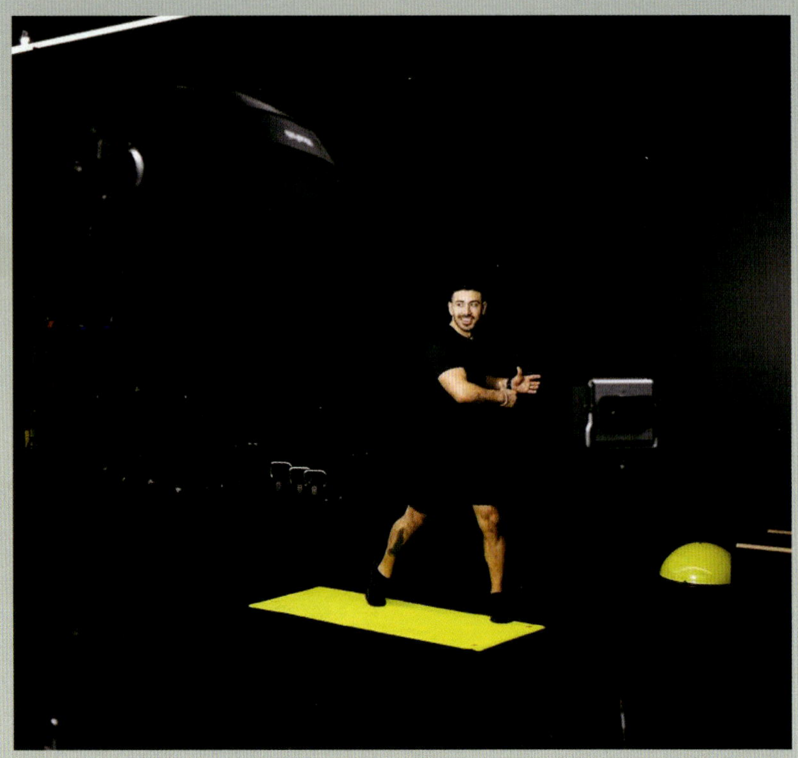

Filming for Acero's online programs was a blast. It's only upwards from here!

finish what was on my plate. Failure to do so wasn't just wasteful, it was positively ungrateful. Yet portion control is one of the reasons that many people put on weight. We simply eat far too much. That's why I encourage my clients to learn how to eat to be satisfied rather than full. But how do you go about that – particularly if it means unlearning the nutritional habits you've developed over a lifetime? It's about developing a more mindful relationship with your daily intake.

NEXT TIME YOU SIT DOWN FOR A MEAL, SCRUTINISE THE FOOD ON YOUR PLATE.

Now consider how much it would take to make you feel full, and then estimate what 80 per cent of that amount would look like. That quantity of food could give you an approximate benchmark as to the amount that could leave you feeling satisfied rather than full.

It's all too easy to wolf down your food almost without thinking, particularly if you're a busy person who eats on the run. Try to slow down. For starters, make sure you're actually sitting down when you eat. Sometimes our stomach fails to register how full it is until the meal is over. Try deliberately eating at a slower pace by consciously savouring the texture and flavours in your mouth, focusing on the sensation as you swallow each forkful. Avoid distractions during your meal times, too, by putting your phone away. This gives you the chance to properly focus on what you're consuming rather than mindlessly chowing down. A study from the University of Rhode Island found that slowing down between bites decreased overall calorie intake by ten per cent.[15]

Also consider whether you are confusing hunger with thirst. Many of us woefully underestimate how much hydration we need. If you stick to a regular intake of three to four litres of water a day, you may be surprised how it affects your appetite and leaves you feeling less ravenous than normal.

For a meal to be satisfy you, it also needs to taste good. A bowl of raw vegetables may be nutritionally sound, but the lack of enjoyment that you'll get from it will probably leave you feeling deprived and hungrily eyeing the dessert trolley. When it comes to breakfast, bacon and eggs is likely to be a far more satisfying meal than a bowl of Rice

Bubbles. In general, high-protein meals will leave you feeling fuller for longer. Bland food can also fail to hit the spot, so use fresh herbs and spices to dial up the flavour and give each mouthful more impact.

UNDERSTANDING MACROS

Unless you're dabbling in keto, try to hit all your macronutrients – protein, fat and carbs – in every single meal. These three nutrients ignite a sense of fullness by releasing hunger-suppressing hormones and raising your blood sugar. If you deprive yourself of them, your body won't feel as satisfied.

Now, as I mentioned, I don't believe a calculator should be a daily part of your culinary toolkit. But it is worth spending a bit of time understanding the proportion of macros you need to hit your specific goals.

CALORIES ARE OBVIOUSLY AN IMPORTANT MEASURE OF YOUR DAILY CONSUMPTION, BUT THEY DON'T ALWAYS GIVE YOU THE FULL PICTURE.

Gram for gram, a handful of mixed nuts might contain more calories that a Curly Wurly – but that doesn't mean chocolate is the better option. When you delve into the macro breakdown, you'll probably find that nuts contain way more protein, less saturated fat and one third of the carbs. The nuts will therefore be better for your hunger and your waistline.

Becoming aware of the nutrient balance can have a big impact on your overall diet. But how can you figure out how to split up your daily macros without the help of a dietician? A macro calculator – they're easy to find online – estimates the macronutrient needs of a person based on their age, physical characteristics, activity level and body weight goals. By plugging in your details, you'll learn the ideal number of calories, and grams of protein, carbs and fat, you need each day.

I don't want you to sit down for every meal with a macro calculator to hand, but I do believe it's worth familiarising yourself with your ideal nutritional breakdown – even if you just track it for a week or two. That knowledge will educate you as to what you should be eating every day.

Most importantly, this approach gives you substantial wiggle room in the type of food you select, as long as it fits into your daily allowance of macros and calories. It liberates you to enjoy your life. Want to meet your mates for a burger? That's fine. Just type it into the macro calculator so you know how many calories you can get away with for the rest of the day to meet your daily goals. Unlike strict diets that put blanket bans on certain forms of deliciousness, this approach allows you to make food choices on the fly, as long as you can shoehorn them into your daily intake.

INTERMITTENT FASTING

Intermittent fasting involves limiting your daily window of eating. Personally, I usually follow a 16:8 timeframe. I'll try to consume all my calories for the day in the eight hours between 10am and 6pm, fasting for the rest of the time – half of which is usually spent fast asleep. There's good reason intermittent fasting has become so fashionable. Essentially, it triggers several changes in your body that make it easier to burn fat by reducing your insulin levels, increasing your growth hormone and slightly boosting your metabolism. A systematic review of 40 studies found that intermittent fasting was effective for weight loss, with adherents typically losing of three to five kilograms over ten weeks.[16]

ANOTHER REASON I LIKE INTERMITTENT FASTING IS THAT IT SIMPLIFIES MY LIFE.

Since the number of hours in which I can indulge is limited I have less room to screw up and cave in to my bad habits and sweet tooth. It stops me from eating late at night – a time when I'm less active and won't be burning off many calories. A recent study showed that the timing of our food intake significantly impacts our energy expenditure and overall appetite.[17] It found that eating later has a profound impact on hunger: the appetite-regulating hormone leptin – which tells the body you're full – decreased for the late-night eaters in the study compared to their earlier-eating counterparts. The late-night group also burned calories at a slower rate. This means you really don't want to be stuffing your face at 10pm.

KNOW YOUR TRIGGERS

Most of us know the fundamental principles of a healthy diet. Familiar nutritional all-stars include fresh fruit and vegetables, wholegrains, lean meats, fish, nuts and dairy. The standard bad guys include a variety of foods high in sugar, salt or saturated fats. We also know that we should watch how much booze we're knocking back, and try to stay within the Australian Government's recommended guidelines by not exceeding ten standard drinks each week.[18] Sure, it might get a bit more nuanced than those principles if you're trying to hit specific fitness or weight-loss goals, but those are the basic cornerstones of a virtuous diet.

Despite knowing the dietary guidelines, most of us struggle to follow them – even when we're feeling motivated to treat ourselves well. Whether our downfall is beer or burgers, glazed doughnuts or gin, our good intentions are constantly derailed by poor decisions and an inability to curb our desires.

SO HOW DO WE OUTSMART THESE NUTRITIONAL SABOTEURS?

For me, the key is to understand the triggers that lead to nutritional transgressions. I've mentioned the benefits of self-tracking already, but it can also prove useful if you're trying to get a handle on a specific vice (and, let's face it, most of us have one). Self-tracking is so helpful because it can help you figure out the emotional or environmental conditions that pre-empt you succumbing to your temptation, which means you can try to find a way to avoid them.

Take booze – the social lubricant on which Australia continues to run – for example. Lots of people drink more than they'd ideally like to. Self-tracking can help you manage your alcohol intake: there are now plenty of apps that can help you track how much booze you're putting away each week. As well as enabling you to keep an eye on your overall consumption and the number of dry days you've had, the data can highlight the occasions when you're susceptible to going too hard. It might be when you catch up with a particular mate for whom 'a couple of drinks' tends to degenerate into rounds of tequila shots. Or it might be when you have to host a dinner with work clients and use alcohol to feel more socially confident.

Whatever your specific alcoholic vulnerability may be, once you've identified those times when your self-control tends to disappear, you can devise a suitable response plan. You might choose to avoid those occasions entirely to remove the source of temptation. Or you might try to offset the damage in the days leading up to the next event by having a few dry days in advance. If you know an occasion is looming where you've been historically prone to overindulgence, you might make a special effort to strengthen your resolve ahead of time. Before you head to a wedding that you know will be awash with booze, take a few minutes beforehand to set your intentions. Perhaps, for example, you might remind yourself of your plan to stick to a set number of drinks before switching to water. You might read some motivational quotes on your phone before you step inside to remind yourself what your goal is and why you're committed to it. Either way, having access to actual data about your boozing should make you more mindful about your relationship with alcohol and the manner in which you drink.

Similarly, if you're struggling to lose weight, keeping a food diary for a period can also be a handy way to figure out where you're going wrong. One weight-loss study found those who kept daily food records lost twice as much weight as those who kept no records.[19] Over a few weeks, note down what you're eating and drinking, how it's prepared, in what quantity and at what time of day or night you consumed it. This will allow you to pinpoint where you're coming unstuck. You might discover, say, that you're diligently nailing your main meals but you're regularly derailed when the midafternoon munchies strike, causing you to hit the office vending machine for a Twix and a bag of chips. Having identified your trigger points you can then work around them – in this case, by bringing a healthy snack to work.

I'm not saying that you have to track every aspect of your life forever. But doing so for a specified timeframe can give you an overarching view of your habits and the intel you need to thrive.

Of course, nutrition is still important and can help with those goals. Do you really understand how your body uses food and manages energy? If you do, you'll find managing your diet will be a little easier. These next couple of sections won't be a replacement for a dietician, but they will help you better plan your diet and fuel your body. You can't lose weight or gain muscle without eating appropriately, so let's get stuck into it!

NUTRIENTS AND THEIR ROLE IN YOUR HEALTH

FATS

Fats are an essential macronutrient, so you need to consume a daily minimum amount of them. While there is a lower limit, though, it's not catastrophic if you drop below this threshold for a short period of time; the detrimental effects of low fat intake will only be apparent after a chronically low intake.

Fats have many important roles in the body, especially in regard to optimising health. They are heavily involved in the production of sex hormones, cell structure, transport and the absorption of fat-soluble vitamins (A, D, E and K).

There are four categories of fats:

- Monounsaturated fats
  - Olive oil, eggs, avocado, and most nuts
- Polyunsaturated fats
  - Salmon, tuna, sardines
- Saturated fats
  - Meat, dairy
- Trans fats
  - Processed and fried foods

Polyunsaturated fats have two subcategories that are considered essential fats and therefore must be consumed throughout the diet. These are omega-6 and omega-3 polyunsaturated fatty acids. These can again be broken into different the following:

- Alpha linoleic acid (omega 3)

- Nuts (especially walnuts), red meat, dairy, flaxseed oil, canola oil

- EPA & DHA (omega 3)
  - Fish and other seafood

- Linoleic Acid (omega 6)

As I mentioned, fats are an essential macronutrient and have a minimum daily average that you need to consume. In general aiming to hit 0.8–1.2 grams per kilogram of body weight is a good target, but you can go as low as 0.5 grams per kilogram of body weight.

Polyunsaturated fats are essential and this means they should obviously be a priority in our diet.

Monounsaturated fats, although not essential, are found in foods that generally have good nutritional quality and so their consumption can definitely be part of a well-balanced diet.

Saturated fat intake will be highly dependent on the source of the food. The aim for saturated fat intake should be to almost exclusively obtain it from meat and dairy products rather than from sweets, pastries and processed foods.

Trans fats for the most part are something we should aim to keep to a minimum in our diet. Trans fats are not naturally occurring fat, as they are created by a manufacturing process called hydrogenation. The human body can't break down this engineered form of fat and therefore it contributes to decreases in high-density lipopotein (HDL) cholesterol (good cholesterol), increases in low-density lipopotein (LDL) cholesterol (bad cholesterol) and increases in inflammation.

What we can gather from all this is that we should aim to obtain our fat intake from almost exclusively natural sources, especially prioritising those foods which provide us with essential polyunsaturated forms. Many of the foods with naturally high occurring fat also contain a solid base of important vitamins and minerals, making them a great inclusion in your diet. While small amounts of fat from processed foods will be fine, chronic overconsumption can lead to some very real health problems.

The other very important factor to consider with fats is their caloric density. Protein and carbs only contain four calories per gram; fats contain nine. This means when equating calories between fats vs carbs or protein, you'd be more than halving the volume of food eaten. This is something to consider when you're looking at satiety, i.e. a high-fat diet may not be appropriate if you're someone who is often hungry. This means while you may be doing the right thing in obtaining all your fats from natural sources, it still must be done in relation to the energy intake that will accompany it. Just like any food or macronutrient, just because it has good properties doesn't mean you can disregard calories when it comes to its consumption, especially fat.

In regards to the timing of your fat consumption, we can look at doing the inverse of our starchy carbs and this is for two reasons.

ONE, THEY DON'T SUPPLY US WITH AN IMMEDIATELY ACCESSIBLE SOURCE OF ENERGY FOR ACTIVITY.

Second, given their structure, they will actually slow the digestion of the other nutrients accompanying them. So, if you consume carbs and protein with a meal high in fats, then digestion will be slower. We want our carbs and protein to be easily digested in the hours surrounding training, and for that reason, maximising your fat intake in times furthest from training is recommended.

Good sources include:

- Avocado
- Oils
- Nuts and seeds
- Cheese
- Milk
- Yoghurt
- Whole eggs
- Salmon

PROTEIN

It's well documented that protein is an essential macronutrient when it comes to building and retaining muscle. You've probably seen people talking about which protein shake is the best, for example. When it comes to body composition and strength-based goals, you would probably consider it one of the essential things to consider alongside resistance training and total calorie intake.

Protein is made up of amino acids. There are 20 amino acids, nine of which the body can't produce itself and as such must be obtained via food. These are known as essential amino acids. A simple way to think about amino acids is that they are the building blocks of protein. We take in protein, the body digests it and converts it into amino acids, and then these amino acids are used in various ways inside the body. They are obviously used for the growth and repair of muscle tissue, but protein also serves roles in the structure and integrity of things like hair and nails.

Protein is also very satiating, meaning it is very filling compared to the other macronutrients. Further, it has a high thermic effect of food (TEF) which means its digestion requires a high amount of energy.

The recommended daily intake (RDI) for protein for those participating in resistance training is between 1.6 g/kg/bw–2.2g/kg/bw. This is due to the recovery demands of muscle from training.

To give us the best chance of muscle gain or retention, we first want to consume enough protein and second we want to evenly spread out this protein intake across our day. The idea behind this is to spend as much time in a state of net muscle protein synthesis (MPS) as possible compared to muscle protein breakdown (MPB). MPS is the creation of new muscle tissue whereas MPB is the breakdown of muscle tissue. These two situations aren't mutually exclusive – they are both always occurring, and so in order to push the ratio in favour of MPS, research has shown it's more beneficial to evenly distribute protein intake across your day. Both protein intake and resistance training stimulate an MPS response. If only protein is ingested, we need to consume 20 grams of protein at a minimum to produce the greatest possible MPS response. Protein intake above this doesn't seem to have any added benefit in the absence of resistance training. Protein requirements when we perform resistance training do however increase. It seems that the threshold beyond which more protein doesn't have an increased effect is now doubled and so the recommended single dose is around 40 grams.

Remember, there are nine essential amino acids that we must consume through food. Meat products contain a full complement of these nine amino acids, whereas many of the non-meat products that are higher in protein don't. This becomes an important factor if you don't eat meat, as it means you must eat a large variety of non-meat-based protein sources to ensure you are getting all nine essential amino acids.

Good sources of protein include:

- Chicken breast
- Lean beef mince

- Pork
- Turkey mince
- Canned tuna
- Egg whites
- Salmon
- Whitefish
- Tofu
- Protein shakes

CARBOHYDRATES

Carbohydrates are our body's most immediate source of energy. Though they are not an 'essential' macronutrient, don't be fooled by influencers talking about the evils of carbs; they're an essential in any balanced diet.

When consumed, they are used immediately for fuel by the body and stored as glycogen in muscle and liver tissue. This stored glycogen is then used when needed by the body. Carbohydrates are our predominant fuel source for activities over 65 per cent in intensity. Lower intensity activities are fuelled mainly by fat, but as the intensity increases, the ratio between carbs and fats begins to switch; high-intensity efforts are almost exclusively fuelled by carbohydrates. For that reason, you can imagine that when it comes to resistance training which is characterised by short, high-intensity efforts, carbohydrates are important.

CARBOHYDRATES WILL HELP FUEL TRAINING SESSIONS, ALLOWING YOU TO TRAIN HARDER.

Adequate carbohydrate intake also helps prevent your body from tapping into protein stores for energy due to its anabolic properties.

Another important factor when looking at carbohydrates is their type. There are two main categories of carbohydrates to consider: simple and complex carbohydrates. Complex carbohydrates can also be broken down into subcategories of fibrous and starchy carbohydrates. The way they are differentiated is by their structure. Simple carbs, as you can probably guess, have a simple structure. This means they are easily broken down and absorbed into the bloodstream. Complex carbs have more intricate structures and therefore are harder for the body to digest. The slower breakdown of complex carbs means that blood glucose has a steadier increase and plateaus after we eat, whereas simple carbs cause a rapid spike in blood glucose. Complex carbs are also generally food which would be characterised as being higher in micronutrients in comparison to simple carbs, meaning the overall nutritional quality is better. Think of complex carbs like your fruits, vegetables and wholegrains, then your simple carbs as being things like chocolate and lollies. For this reason, as a general rule of thumb, it's best to keep most of your carbs coming from complex sources and only a small amount from simple carbs. Carbohydrates are a huge category of food, and you might be surprised to learn that fruit and vegetables are also classified as carbohydrates alongside the more obvious grain and wheat-based products. This is where we get into the subcategories of complex carbohydrates.

When we say that carbohydrates are a non-essential macronutrient, all that this means is that they don't need to be consumed through your diet in order to be found in the body. This is because when energy is needed, fats and protein can be converted into glucose and used for energy. With that being said, carbohydrates should make up a large portion of our diet. Essentially, once you have met the protein and fat requirements for your goal, carbohydrates can fill in the rest.

Now, given we know carbohydrates are such a diverse food group and the effects they have on our body are largely dependent on their structure, we can pick from the categories of carbohydrates to help make decisions as to which type suits our needs.

These categories are:

- Fibrous carbohydrates
- Starchy carbohydrates
- Simple carbohydrates

Fibrous carbohydrates have higher fibre content and this means they have a low-calorie density. Essentially, you'll be able to eat large volumes for fewer calories, and this becomes particularly important for those in a fat loss phase. Higher fibre foods are also important for digestion and general gut health.

Fibrous carbs include:

- Leafy greens
- Broccoli
- Green beans
- Peas
- Cabbage
- Carrots

- Zucchini
- Celery
- Mushrooms
- Apples
- Blueberries
- Strawberries

It's easiest to consider these in relation to servings of fruit and vegetables. For most people, 1–3 servings of fruit and 2–5 servings of vegetables is ideal no matter what your calorie target is. The reason I've measured in servings of fruit and vegetables and not just fibre is because fruits and vegetables are very high in micronutrients; only focusing on fibre intake can mean you don't get all the key micronutrients that fruit and vegetables supply.

Both starchy and fibrous carbohydrates are considered complex carbohydrates. The main difference between the two is the fibre content, which in turn changes how they interact with the body when consumed. Given the fibre content is lower, starchy carbs are generally more calorie-dense and are broken down and absorbed into the bloodstream faster.

Starchy carbs are the preferred way in which we get energy for exercise and daily activity. Both starchy and simple carbohydrates would be considered the main players when it comes to providing energy, but in general, starchy carbohydrates have a better nutritional value. This is why their intake is preferrable for fuelling our body for exercise and daily activities. Aiming to obtain your carbohydrate and energy intake through fibrous carbohydrates would be extremely hard given their high fibre content, and this is why they are in their own category. When looking to structure your nutrition plan, although they are both complex carbs, you should consider fibrous carbohydrates and starchy carbohydrates separately as they both have quite distinct roles.

Examples of starchy carbs include:

- Bread
- Pasta
- Rice (both brown and white)
- Potatoes
- Bananas
- Pumpkin
- Cous cous
- Muesli

Lastly, we have simple carbohydrates. As we know, they have simple structures that mean they are easily absorbed into the bloodstream. We also discussed that, along with starchy carbohydrates, simple carbohydrates' role when consumed will be to provide energy. Basically, you get a big hit of calories for little amounts of food volume, which makes them great for energy but also very easy to overconsume. This can come in handy, though: if you are massing and struggling with increasing your food intake, adding in some simple carbohydrates may help you hit your prescribed targets without making you feel sick.

In summary, everyone should include fibrous carbohydrates in their everyday nutrition as they are major players in our general health, and spreading them evenly across all your meals during the day is good practice. In regards to energy intake, both starchy and simple carbohydrates will do the job, but it's best practice to heavily bias starchy carbohydrates for their increased nutritional value. Also given that these carbohydrates are largely responsible for energy and then replenishment of used energy, biasing their intake pre, during and post-workout has been shown to be beneficial.

AN OVERVIEW OF MACRONUTRIENTS AND HOW THEY RELATE TO BODY COMPOSITION

Energy balance essentially dictates changes in our total mass, i.e. if we are in a surplus, we will gain mass and if we are in a deficit, lose mass. Which mass (fat or muscle) changes can be manipulated by how we structure our intake of macronutrients, specifically protein.

As we now know, there are three main macronutrients:

- Protein
- Carbs
- Fats

Protein is essentially the building block of muscle tissue and therefore adequate intake of protein is important for growth and retention. When you think about body composition the goal is to increase muscle mass and reduce fat mass.

As it relates to fat loss, the goal is to maintain muscle mass we have previously built and at the same time lose fat. Outside regular resistance training, protein intake will have a large bearing on whether we achieve fat loss or weight loss. Weight loss is simply just the loss of mass no matter where it's from. If all you did was eat under your maintenance calories then without resistance training or a high protein intake you would lose fat AND muscle. Muscle is energetically costly to the body and therefore if it's not being used then it will atrophy. While in a deficit, if we keep training and ensure we are eating sufficient protein, we are providing a stimulus sufficient enough to ensure muscle mass is maintained but fat is lost.

In regards to increasing muscle mass, again, sufficient protein intake is important. Given you would be in calorie surplus when looking to increase weight, there is a little more wiggle room in terms of protein intake, and we don't necessarily need to have as high an intake as we would in a deficit.

In terms of body composition, carbs and fats are important, but have less of a direct impact compared to protein intake, so measuring specific amounts of each is less important.

COMMON NUTRITION MYTHS AND MISCONCEPTIONS

Calories In, Calories Out (CICO) Is All That Matters

CICO is a powerful tool for many people as it allows them to move away from chasing the next fad diet or trying to avoid certain foods or whole food groups, all while still achieving their goals. However, though energy balance is the only thing that will directly cause changes in weight and yes, you could potentially achieve your goals by just eating 'junk' food, does that mean you should?

PROBABLY NOT.

Here are some main examples of why:

- Keeping protein intake high is important for muscle gain and retention
- Fat has a minimum intake for hormonal purposes
- You're likely missing out on many important micronutrients which are generally not found in a diet consisting of 'junk' food
- Given these foods are highly calorie-dense and palatable they make control over their consumption difficult

In summary, while CICO is the driver of your changes in body composition, it's highly recommended that you do so with good nutritional habits and nutritious foods.

Calories In, Calories Out Is Irrelevant

Yes, you read correctly! There is a large cohort of called coaches and experts who believe when it comes to body composition, things like hormones, gut health and other factors will override the principle of energy balance.

Statements such as 'You'll never lose fat if your (insert hormone) is always low' or 'Your gut microbiome is damaged, that's why you struggle to lose fat' are common examples of what you may hear. Generally, these statements are followed by 'Buy my product to fix it'.

Now, while paying attention to hormone levels and gut health is actually good practice, it will never break the law of the energy balance. Yes, there are other factors that may inhibit your ability to create that deficit and it may be important to address them ... but if you're not losing fat, then you aren't in an energy deficit.

Carbohydrates Make You Fat

The word 'carbohydrates' can essentially be interchanged with any other specific food or macronutrient. No one single food or macronutrient will cause you to gain weight. Again, energy balance is the key factor you must always remember. So, when someone says 'I took carbs out of my diet and lost weight', this may be true but it's because they took out calories (which come from carbohydrates). The same thing would have happened if they took out fat or even protein. It's very well documented that when calories are equated, there is no one 'best' diet for fat loss (unless under certain medical conditions).

Don't Eat Before Bed

This is derived from the thought that because we are inactive at night, consuming calories before we sleep will means there is a heap of energy that we will not use and therefore store as fat. Firstly, your body never stops using energy and there are many important metabolic processes occurring while we are asleep. But again, energy balance is the key factor here and this will be the defining factor in changes in weight, not when you eat food.

Starvation Mode

A term that has gathered some momentum in recent times is 'starvation mode'. Like many of the other new age terms floating around the fitness industry, it lacks substance and generally has a very simple explanation.

The idea of 'starvation mode' basically revolves around the idea that at some point, when your body is subject to a lengthy dieting period or low-calorie intake, your body will halt fat loss in order to survive.

BASICALLY, NO MATTER WHAT THIS PERSON DOES, THEY CAN'T LOSE FAT.

While the concept does have some truth to it, a better understanding of the actual mechanisms at hand would allow people to put actions in place to ensure future fat loss success. The part of starvation mode that holds true is that your body will respond to periods of time in an energy deficit, and after long enough, there will be a point where that calorie deficit will no longer yield results. This is actually a well-known mechanism within the body called 'adaptive thermogenesis'. This is a natural process your body will implement in order to restore the balance between energy coming into the body vs energy going out.

The underlying principle that will dictate successful fat loss is calorie deficit. If you don't know what that is, basically the amount of energy we expel day to day, week to week must be more than what we consume day to day and week to week. In a calorie deficit your body will mobilise stored fat in order to produce energy needed to survive and function. Outside external intervention (surgery) there is no other way to lose fat and if you are in a calorie deficit for a long enough period of time, there is no way you won't lose fat.

UP YOUR SATIETY GAME FOR FAT LOSS SUCCESS

We all know that hunger is a bi-product of dieting for fat loss. In a prolonged energy deficit with the aim of losing fat, you should expect that at some stage a level of hunger will develop and it's something that you will have to consistently deal with on the path to a leaner physique. Let's be honest, dieting would be a breeze for everyone if hunger wasn't an issue. In terms of addressing hunger, eating to satiety is the obvious answer ... which of course is not always conducive to fat loss.

You could wrap an internal band around your gut to help, but I don't recommend it (unless medically it's been advised). This makes things a bit tricky. Feeling hungry and craving food is a large part of why so many fat loss diets fail. Our bodies don't like being in a net energy deficit and therefore it will do a number of things physiologically to get you out of that deficit. Combine this with psychological factors that arise from that same deficit, and you find yourself in a situation where every bone in your body is telling you to eat until you are full and sometimes even further!

SO HOW CAN WE MITIGATE THE EFFECTS OF HUNGER?

Well, aside from cognitive restraint and some determination to reach your goal, we can increase satiation.

Satiety is defined is 'the feeling of fullness after a meal', while satiation is 'the end of the desire to eat'. Satiety is somewhat of a 'diet hack'. We see people quite regularly advocating for eating any foods you want that fit your macros or, more specifically, any of the yummy tasty foods you want. While the underlying concept is not wrong as you're still aiming for a calorie deficit, maintaining this proves hard in most cases. Why? If the goal is to fit as much so-called 'junk' food into our prescribed macros, the thing that will catch up to the majority of us is hunger. It's all well and good to enjoy eating palatable foods when dieting, but be prepared to be hungry. The reason being is that many of these foods are what you'd categorise as calorie-dense. This means for the volume of food you ingest, the calorie content is relatively high, and while you may enjoy your meal, you'll likely be left hungry. Further, highly palatable foods are designed to make you want to go back for more as they generally have high sugar and fat contents. If you instead temporarily sacrifice the need to eat these tasty palatable foods for more filling foods, your dieting experience might require much less cognitive restraint to see you through to the end.

Halt et al. produced a satiety index (SI) of 38 common foods. They found that boiled potatoes had an SI of 323 per cent compared to white bread, being the reference food with an SI of 100 per cent. They found that in general, the serving size was the strongest predictor of SI.

There is a vast array of food outside of the 38 foods listed, which will also provide high ratings on the satiety index: lean proteins such as steak and chicken, and numerous vegetables and fruits. Foods that are highly satiating are what we categorise as having a low-calorie density.

ESSENTIALLY, YOU CAN EAT LARGE VOLUMES OF THAT FOOD FOR A SMALLER NUMBER OF CALORIES.

These foods generally include one or more of the following:

- High protein
- High fibre
- High water content
- Generally less fat

Eating these types of foods will result in large, bulky meals containing low calories. The ability to eat these volumes of food triggers gastric distention, which enables the stomach to send signals to the brain to recognise satiety. Highly palatable small meals, on the other hand, won't have the same desired effect. With satiation being so low with the aforementioned meal, the desire to eat again sooner will ultimately make your dieting experience that much harder to deal with.

HOW THE BODY MANAGES ENERGY

Flexible Dieting & IIFYM (If It Fits Your Macros) are concepts you've likely heard floating around the health and fitness industry in the last decade. Essentially, they're the idea that you can eat whatever you want within a calorie allowance and still achieve your body composition goals. Yes, you can eat burgers, doughnuts, Maccas … all the good stuff and still lose weight.

Of course, we should know by now that it's not that simple. The human body doesn't like being in an energy deficit. It would much rather have balance, the right amount of energy coming in for what it expends. For that reason, when we reduce our food (a.k.a. energy intake) the body will find ways to reduce energy output and even try to increase energy input.

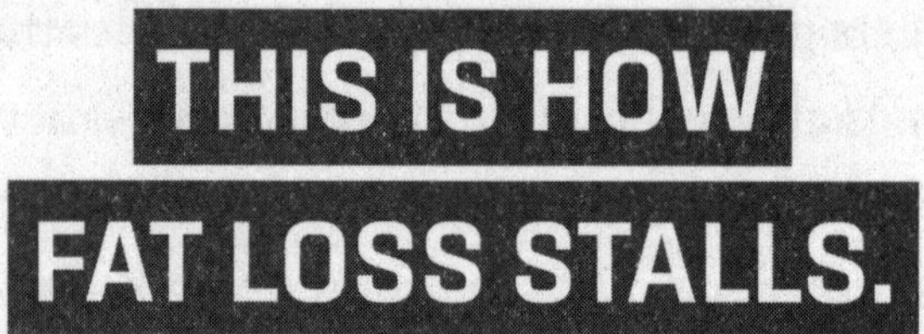

But why? How? Let's take a look.

Basal Metabolic Rate (BMR)

All systems and metabolic processes in the body require energy. BMR essentially refers to the sum of these energy outputs when our body is at complete rest.

In order to conserve energy, the body will begin to lower the output of some of these systems and become more efficient. Firstly, the bigger the individual, the more energy the body requires to 'keep the lights on'. If you lose weight, you are carrying less weight and therefore you cost less to run, hence a decrease in your body's BMR.

But this can go badly if it happens for too long, and your body will start to shut down key processes. For example, when people with uteruses have been extensively dieting for an extended length of time, they will lose their menstrual cycle: survival has become the body's current priority, not reproduction. This may sound great if your menstrual cycle is particularly painful, but it's actually a bad thing and a sign that your body is very, very stressed. And of course, we now know that the body will halt fat loss if you diet too hard for too long – balance and a long-term plan is key.

Non Exercise Activity Thermogenesis (NEAT)

NEAT is the amount of energy you burn from your day-to-day unplanned activity. To paint the picture, a construction worker whose job requires manual labour is going to have much higher NEAT than an admin worker who sits at a desk all day. When an individual diets, reductions in their NEAT become a huge reason why progress stalls. Basically, your body will respond to the deficit by making you move less. You will sit at every opportunity, take the car instead of walking and even fidget less. Some people even speak slower. All of this reduces energy output, and is the body's way to offset the deficit that you have created through eating less food.

Exercise Activity (EA)

This is the energy burned from planned exercise. A key thing to consider here is that while you don't want this to drop, it also doesn't burn as many calories as people think. This means that if you purely try to exercise your way to fat loss, you're taking a very inefficient approach.

Another reason why using exercise as your main driver of creating an energy deficit is not a great idea is because you can't really accurately track how many calories you are burning (despite what tech companies like to think, your treadmill and watch are not that accurate). Tracking food may not be perfect, but is a much more reliable and effective approach.

Thermic Effect of Food (TEF)

The thermic effect of food basically states that the process of digesting food requires energy and some foods require more energy to digest than others. Eating less, as required in a diet, will mean the amount of energy expended digesting food will be less. Consuming high-protein and fibrous foods will help offset this reduction as much as possible.

With all these physiological factors in effect, it would be remiss of us not to mention we also have a psychological drive to eat more. That is being hungry all the time and a higher perceived food focus. But we won't go too far into that rabbit hole.

As you can see from that overview, fat loss is a constant fight between you and your body. You create a deficit and lose fat but at the same time your body is making adaptions that eventually mean you will no longer be in a deficit. What this tells us is that it's not impossible to keep losing fat, but it can become more difficult and even harmful if not done properly.

In terms of addressing adaptive thermogenesis, you first need to ensure you are actually creating a calorie deficit with your food. Do you actually know how many calories you should be eating and if so are you actually sticking to those calories consistently? If you can't answer 'yes' to both of those questions then that is where you need to start first.

Say you were on the money with your calories and after three weeks of losing fat, you have plateaued. What can you do from there? You need to again tip that energy in VS energy out equation back in favour of energy out. From an energy in perspective it's relatively straightforward, decrease your calories. In terms of energy out, we need to look at the systems above that expel energy. In summary:

BMR

There are probably no mechanisms or strategies you can use to increase BMR or maintain it while dieting.

TEF

With food intake decreasing, TEF will also decrease but you can do your best to keep it as high as possible by eating plenty of protein and fibre.

EA

As I mentioned, you shouldn't be trying to 'exercise' your way to a deficit. It's very inefficient. In terms of training, we recommend you aim to maintain similar levels as to what you were performing previous to your cut.

NEAT

Natural decreases in NEAT as we diet can quickly bring progress to a halt if not monitored. This is often a big reason to why you hear people say 'I am so strict with my calories but I am not losing weight'; their NEAT has dropped drastically.

HITTING PLATEAUS AND HOW TO MOVE FORWARD

So we have determined that 'starvation mode' is essentially a misinterpreted version of adaptive thermogenesis. We also know now that adaptive thermogenesis will create stalls in progress that can be addressed by decreasing calorie intake or increasing energy expenditure. Now, as you keep decreasing calories and increasing expenditure to address these fat loss stalls, there is going to eventually come a time where it is no longer viable or sustainable.

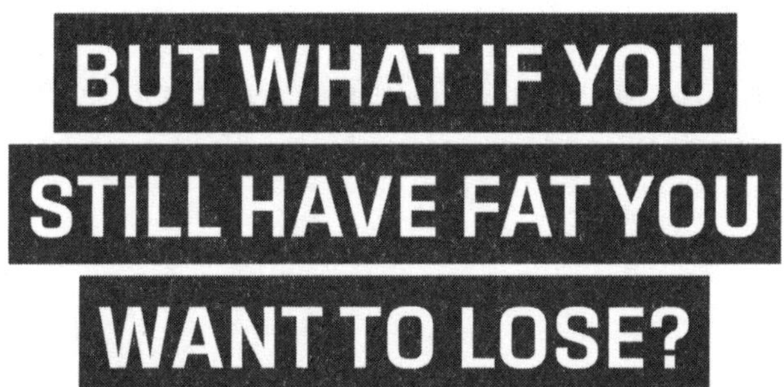

A prime example is someone that has yo-yo dieted for years now finds themselves in a position where they have fat they want to lose but are maintaining on very low calories. They will make initial changes that will result in a small loss, but very quickly they will get to a place where their calories are very low, activity is very high, and they just can't push it anymore. But again, the reason that fat loss is not occurring isn't because it can't – it 100 per cent can. It's because the calorie deficit that is required is very hard to achieve, and is likely unsafe or simply not viable.

This is a tricky position to be in. It may be time to reassess your relationship with food and your body, especially if you have a history of yo-yo dieting. Do you really need to lose that weight? Or is this a mental block rather than an issue of physical health? We know that disordered eating can closely tie to the desire to lose weight, so it's important to check in with yourself.

If it is a matter of wanting to lose more fat, you'll likely need a reverse or recovery diet to set yourself up for future fat loss. This is something I strongly recommend you see a dietician for, as what you'll need will be specific to your body and medical history.

KEY TAKEAWAYS

On the surface, the concept of simply adhering to a calorie target with whatever foods you like seems relatively straightforward. Anyone who has dieted will tell you it doesn't generally work that way. While it may be doable, it would come with a cost. You have to ask yourself, is it really worth spending all that time being hungry, craving more food and fighting the good fight to remain in cognitive control of your food consumption? Or is the temporary sacrifice of stepping away from the most palatable foods in a bid to increase your satiety during a diet more worth your while?

If you are the outlier that can resist the temptation to eat during extreme hunger for weeks on end as long as you get your food fix, then go for it. But for the majority of the population, this won't cut it. I know for a fact that I would rather feel full during the length of a diet than have a burger each day. Opting for foods and structuring meals on the high end of the satiety index will help you remain fuller for longer and in turn, help you to navigate the harshness of dieting.

MY PERSONAL **TRANSFORMATION**

A little aside, here. You might be thinking, *but Jono, it's easy for you to talk about nutrition and losing a lot of weight - you don't know how hard it is!* (This may be especially if you've seen some of my photos floating around on Instagram). But I *do* know. I haven't always been a shining paragon of muscular vigour propelled by drop sets, green smoothies and early nights. There was one period when my life careered out of control.

Divorce is invariably heartbreaking and complicated. I'd been with Amy since I was 16 years old and by the time we split I was 31. That was the entirety of my adult life. Amy knew me inside out - she knew what I was thinking without me even saying a word. When we first met I was still a skinny teenager chasing my soccer dream. Since then we'd been on a journey together, building our joint business that slowly grew to include the Acero gym and fitness app. Today Amy and I continue to work closely together. She's still the backbone of our business and I trust her completely.

All of this is a longwinded way of saying that, when we finally split in 2022, my head was all over the place. It was such a confusing time for me, personally and professionally. Part of it was that I felt like such a failure; but I'd also never been through such emotional upheaval. There were all these conflicting feelings bouncing through my brain - fear, uncertainty, anxiety, rage. I was a total mess. It was the lowest point in my life.

People handle divorce in different ways. Some turn to drink or drugs to numb the pain. Some rebound into wildly inappropriate relationships. Some get nasty and find themselves stuck in bitter custody battles over who gets to keep the Le Creuset casserole set.

I SET ABOUT SUBCONSCIOUSLY TRYING TO SABOTAGE MY CAREER.

A big part of it was how I looked after myself - basically, I stopped completely. Something weird happened to me mentally where I just couldn't make myself train anymore. Looking back I suspect I may have been depressed; it was like I'd lost all my enthusiasm for life. One way this manifested was through a form of extreme physical lethargy. I couldn't even summon the energy to do ten push-ups.

Training has always been my go-to strategy to maintain my mental equilibrium. Exercise is my number-one source of stress relief. It straightens out my head and makes me feel better in body and mind. So without that positive influence in my life, I started to seek out those mood-boosting endorphins in less positive places. I turned to alcohol and partying to try to escape my miserable headspace. After years of being nutritionally disciplined I embraced fast food in a big, big way. McDonald's, Mad Mex, Oporto - I ate whatever I wanted whenever I could.

I felt so desperate that I decided I needed to escape Sydney, so I went on a long holiday to party in Vegas, New York and Mexico. Needless to say this wasn't the most responsible move as a business owner. I didn't say goodbye to anyone and I was gone for three whole months. The business took a hit while I basically left everyone at the gym working their arses off while I went AWOL and tried to distract myself with some fun. Looking back, I think a lot of people who worked for me lost their trust in me at that stage. I can hardly blame them. While all this was going on, I also stopped posting anything on Instagram. That might not sound like a big deal, but my social media profile has played a big role in my career. I was neglecting that as well.

It's scary when I think about it now, but I didn't do a single workout for almost six months. Obviously that had a dramatic physical effect. I put on about 20 kilograms, which put me up to 108 kilograms. My belly got so big that I could balance a beer on it. The worst thing was that, as a trainer with a reasonable profile, how you look really does matter. If a personal trainer can't look after themselves, who's going to trust them to oversee their own training? My professional credibility was on the line. Let's just say that I embraced baggy t-shirts in a very big way!

WHAT HAPPENED NEXT WAS MY LUCKY BREAK.

I'd been the trainer for Australian *Men's Health* for a couple of years at this stage and was good friends with the editor at the time, Scott Henderson. As I've described in this book, I'd overseen a few celebrity transformations for the magazine - training stars into cover-model shape in 12 weeks. When Scott saw the sorry state that I'd got myself into, he was like, 'Whoa!' I was a little worried that *Men's Health* might give me the elbow, but instead Scott had the vision to spot an opportunity. 'Why don't you do your own 12-week transformation?' he suggested. 'Then we could make the cover about you.'

That was such a big moment for me. Something I've always done at the beginning of each year is to sit down and write out my personal goals for the next 12 months. For the past decade, one thing had always been on my list: to appear on the cover of *Men's Health*. When Scotty dangled that opportunity in front of me, it was like a switch was flicked in my head.

I instantly rediscovered my sense of purpose. Until that moment I'd lost my passion for training and surrendered my motivation. Worse, I felt I'd lost my team's faith and could no longer inspire my clients in the way I previously had. The positive energy that I'd always prided myself on wasn't there, because it seemed hypocritical to preach to people about health and fitness, when I couldn't even look after myself. The underlying purpose behind my transformation wasn't only about trying to look ripped on the cover. It was about trying to regain my self-respect and the confidence of all these people that I felt I'd let down.

LOSING THE BOOZE

I had 12 weeks to lose about 20 kilograms and get myself in shape for the *Men's Health* cover. Failing to nail this opportunity would be personally devastating and professionally humiliating. In short, I couldn't afford to fuck it up!

The first thing I did was stop drinking. I gave my sozzled liver a much-needed break after the hammering it'd copped since the split. This decision was a no-brainer for multiple reasons - the most obvious being that alcohol is high in calories, contributing to weight that I urgently needed to shed. Plus I've always found that I'm more likely to make bad dietary decisions once I've had a couple of drinks. I either overeat or choose less healthy options. I mean, have you ever eaten a kebab while sober?

The other reason was that I needed my metabolism to be firing on all cylinders. Booze derails that process because it contains ethanol which is a fairly toxic substance. When your liver is confronted by a few drinks it takes a safety-first approach and prioritises breaking down ethanol into by-products that can be used or flushed out of the body. With its attention diverted to this pressing task, the liver slows down the body's metabolism of fat, storing it in your cells instead. Bottom line: margaritas were incompatible with my need to get in shape fast.

FAST MOVES

I also began a process of intermittent fasting whereby I consumed all my daily food in an eight-hour window between 10am and 6pm. Ultimately, I knew that *what* I ate was always going to be more important than *when* I ate it. I still find intermittent fasting a helpful strategy for weight loss, though; along with reducing insulin levels, it also gives me less room to screw up. It gives me a firm cut-off time and stops me from snacking at night, so I consume fewer calories overall.

PLATE EXPECTATIONS

When it came to my diet, I knew I had to find a food plan that would be sustainable enough for me to actually stick to it. Twelve weeks is a reasonable stint of time and I knew that the longer I could maintain a diet of nutritious foods, the more benefits I'd reap.

Too often I've seen clients try to maintain a crazy-strict diet. They might manage to follow it for a week or two, before they understandably go rogue. I know from training thousands of people that if you can stick to a dietary or exercise plan for four weeks, you'll start to see proper results. But that means the plan needs to be realistic.

Essentially, my plan was simply to eat three meals per day. I didn't count my calories; I just focused on getting all my macronutrients in every meal. The percentage ratio I tried to stick to on my plate was 40 per cent protein, 40 per cent carbs and 20 per cent fat. The beauty of that plan was its simplicity. Beyond that I just ate to be satisfied (within reason), and as soon as I was satiated, I put down my fork. That plan might sound basic, but I knew that if I stuck to it and trained hard enough, it would do the trick.

FASTED CARDIO

During my 12-week challenge, five days a week I'd do some form of fasted cardio. Each morning I'd usually jump on a StairMaster treadmill and keep walking until I'd burned 300 calories, or do the cardio equivalent on another machine.

I like fasted cardio as a weight-loss tactic because, when you're exercising in this state, your body preferentially burns fat for energy, as your blood sugar and insulin levels are low due to your empty stomach. Consequently it's a good way to try to lower your body-fat percentage. Be warned, however, if you try to stick to fasted cardio long-term your body will adapt, like with any type of long-term exercise routine. Switch it up every few weeks to keep it effective.

TRAIN AND GAIN

In addition to my fasted cardio, I committed to training five times a week for between 45 minutes and an hour. I would target a different muscle group every day. I was chasing a form of hypertrophy by working each specific muscle group to failure, attacking it with three related exercises performed back-to-back with only one minute's rest in between sets. Here's how my program looked:

MONDAY

CHEST

1a Bench press × 12
1b Cable flies × 12
1c Dips × 12

Perform the three exercises back-to-back then rest for one minute. Repeat five times.

TUESDAY

BACK

1a Barbell overarm rows × 12
1b Barbell underarm rows × 12
1c Straight-arm cable pullover × 12

Perform the three exercises back-to-back then rest for one minute. Repeat five times.

WEDNESDAY

LEGS

1a Leg extensions × 12
1b Barbell squats × 12
1c Dumbbell lunges × 12

Perform the three exercises back-to-back then rest for one minute. Repeat five times.

THURSDAY

SHOULDERS

1a Dumbbell shoulder press × 12
1b Dumbbell lateral raises × 12
1c Dumbbell front raises × 12

Perform the three exercises back-to-back then rest for one minute. Repeat five times.

FRIDAY

BICEPS

1a Underarm barbell curls × 12
1b Overarm barbell curls × 12
1c Dumbbell hammer × 12

Perform the three exercises back-to-back then rest for one minute. Repeat five times.

TRICEPS

1a Triceps pushdown with rope × 12
1b Triceps overhead extension with rope × 12
1c Dumbbell skull crushes × 12

Perform the three exercises back-to-back then rest for one minute. Repeat five times.

At the end of each workout I'd do an eight-minute circuit where I'd alternate cardio with some form of core work. For example, I'd jump on the Assault Bike for 30 seconds and then do 30 seconds of sit-ups, then repeat. Doing that really gets the heart pumping.

In addition, every night I'd try to go for a 30-minute walk at a gentle pace. In part that was to try to get a few more steps in, but it was mainly to unwind and relax. I live in Bondi and the surrounding coast is beautiful, so I found the walk was a valuable form of stress release that helped me chill out before I hit the hay. I prioritised my sleep, too - making sure I got at least eight hours every single night.

MINDSET

Twelve weeks is a fair old stint - 84 days of hard work, sacrifice and self-denial. To make it seem more manageable, I broke it down in my head into four-week blocks and focused on getting the best possible results in each of them.

What I've learned with my clients is that if you stick at something for four weeks, you can really notice aesthetic results that you'll never get after just one or two weeks. Breaking it down into those subgoals kept me motivated and made it more achievable, too. I also took photos of myself in the mirror each week to track my progress along the way. Seeing small improvements encouraged me that I really was on the right track.

THE RESULTS

After 12 long weeks I finished the challenge having lost 17 kilograms. That was a lot of weight I no longer had to haul around my gut, and I felt lighter mentally too. The transformation was almost like a form of redemption. After such a dark episode in my life when I felt so lost and directionless, I'd regained control and recovered the man I wanted to be.

I didn't see the cover pictures until the big reveal party that we held at Acero. About 100 people were there - my gym colleagues, my friends and my family. Crucially, Amy was there, too. We turned the boxing ring into a makeshift stage and I got up there with Ben Jhoty, the new *Men's Health* editor, who pulled back a sheet to reveal a life-size version of the cover.

Standing up there and seeing that cover was an emotional experience. I'd been on other magazine covers, from *Fitness First* to *Men's Fitness*, but this one felt special. Because I'd had to work so much harder to make this physical comeback, somehow it felt more meaningful.

One moment stands out above any others from that night. My dad is an old-school Colombian man of few words. He's endured a hard life at times, but just soldiers on through his challenges and rarely grumbles. Being from that background and the generation he was born into, he isn't very comfortable expressing his emotions. But at one point that evening, he came up to me and whispered in my ear.

'You know,' he said, 'I'm really proud of you, Jono.'

Dad had never expressed anything like that to me before. For me, that really meant a lot.

PILLAR 4

SLEEP

'You snooze, you lose' would have to be one of the most inaccurate phrases in the known universe. Nothing could be further from the truth. Most people neglect sleep. We've become seduced by the #grindset mentality that we should all be striving to outwork the competition by waking at the crack of dawn and logging superhuman hours before spending any leftover time on some half-baked side hustle.

Whether you're an early bird or a night owl, sleep is your secret weapon. Ensuring you get regular quality shut-eye might not sound very dynamic or exciting, but prioritising sleep could be the key to making yourself sharper, leaner, stronger, healthier and far less miserable all-round.

Admittedly I do get up heinously early in the morning: my alarm clock usually goes off by 4am at the latest, and my first session with a client is often at 4.30am. But to make that sustainable, I'll usually go to bed at 8pm. That's not very rock'n'roll is it? Yet I've learned that without a solid eight hours of sleep, I'm not as mentally alert or present at work – essentially I'm a second-rate version of myself. I honestly believe that the quality of my sleep determines the outcome of my entire day. Going to bed early does mean that I sometimes miss out on certain things. But looking at the evidence, this is a sacrifice I need to make.

IF YOU HAVE FITNESS OR WEIGHT-LOSS GOALS, ENSURING YOU'RE GETTING ENOUGH KIP COULD BE THE DECISIVE FACTOR THAT MAKES THE DIFFERENCE BETWEEN SUCCESS AND FAILURE.

The science behind that view is emphatic.

COMPETITIVE ADVANTAGE

Forget doping to improve performance. Sports scientists have long known that sleep can give athletes the winning edge. Back in 2011, scientists at Stanford University published a study to explore the tangible benefits of catching extra Z's.[20] They took 11 players from the Stanford University men's basketball team, who committed to getting ten hours of sleep a night during the study period. The knock-on effect of extra sleep on their sporting performance was phenomenal. The players not only started to run faster in both half-court and full-court sprints, their shooting also improved by at least nine per cent. Those are staggering results in a world that's all about securing marginal gains.

Not surprisingly, the rest of the sporting world has since caught on to this relatively simple way of getting an advantage. Soccer teams Manchester United, Chelsea and Real Madrid have recruited sleep coaches to help their players zonk out more effectively. The teams' sports scientists know that, just like nutrition and hydration, sleep is a vital contributor to an athlete's physical conditioning, physiological recovery and performance. Many top clubs have even incorporated sleeping pods into their facilities. These specially designed bedrooms enable players to make tactical visits to snoozeville between training sessions.

BEING SLEEP DEPRIVED WILL AFFECT HOW YOU FARE IN THE GYM EVEN IF YOU'RE NOT AN ELITE ATHLETE.

One study found that inadequate rest impairs your muscle strength in compound movements.[21] The beauty of sleep is that, unlike costly supplements, it's absolutely free. When you want to build muscle mass, you're undermining your efforts if you're not prioritising your sleep.

SLEEP AND WEIGHT LOSS

Sleep can alter your body composition in the other direction, too. How long you spend in the land of nod can determine whether or not you're above your healthy weight. One study found that people who regularly slept fewer than six hours per night were far more likely to have excess body weight, while people who got an average of eight hours per night had the lowest relative body fat of the study group.[22]

If you're trying to shed weight, insufficient sleep could prove as disastrous to your goal as getting a job in a cake shop. One study found that people trying to slim down by following a low-calorie diet achieved the same amount of weight loss irrespective of whether they slept for an average of 5.5 or 8.5 hours per night.[23] When it delved deeper, however, the study found that for those who slept under six hours, a significantly higher proportion of the weight they lost came from lean mass (muscle) instead of fat. For that sleep-deprived group, only a quarter of the weight loss came from fat, while those who got 8.5 hours of sleep lost twice as much fat.

Aside from affecting their weight loss, a lack of sleep was also bad news for the participants' self-control. In the experiment, both groups were supposed to eat the same amount of food. But those who slept less made up for it with knife and fork, guzzling more than 300 extra calories the following day. The reason for this, the researchers believed, is that lack of sleep causes a spike in ghrelin (the hormone that makes you feel hungry) accompanied by a fall in leptin (the hormone that signals your brain that you feel full).

MENTAL CLARITY

If you feel a bit foggy after a poor night's sleep, you're not imagining things. Your attention and concentration abilities are proven to decline with a lack of sleep, while your reaction time also slows down[24]. That might affect your chances of winning a game of ping-pong or the time it takes you to complete Wordle, but there are far more serious repercussions, too.

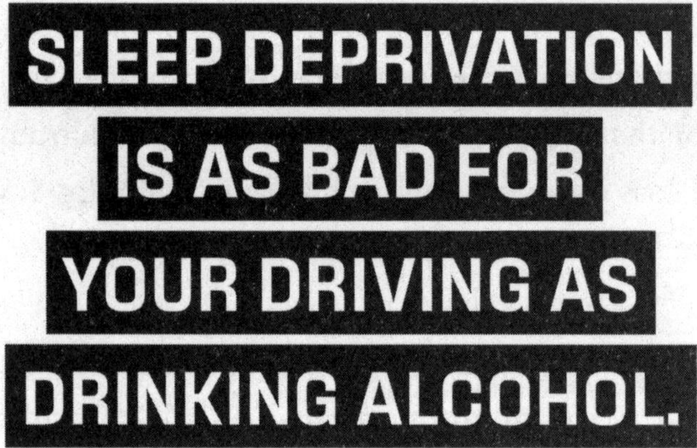

Going without sleep for 48 hours impairs cognitive abilities to the same degree as having a blood alcohol concentration of 0.1 per cent.[25] It's a question that's worth asking after you've pulled an all-nighter: are you too tired to drive? If you are, you also probably shouldn't be lifting heavy weights at the gym – maintaining technique requires serious concentration, particularly for riskier movements like squatting barbells. Sometimes the best thing you can do for your body is take a day off and do lighter exercise like cardio or walking, and try to rest. You won't lose your gains overnight!

THE MOODY BLUES

My mate's wise mum has a saying: 'The difference between hope and despair is a good night's sleep.' She's onto something, too. You've probably experienced the way in which a bad night's sleep affects your outlook. It can make you feel more crotchety and less emotionally resilient. You don't have to stay up all night to cop those negative effects, either: even partial sleep deprivation can have a big impact on your mood. Researchers from the University of Pennsylvania found that participants who were limited to only 4.5 hours of sleep a night for one week reported feeling more stressed, angry, sad and mentally exhausted.[26] As soon as they resumed normal sleep patterns they reported a dramatic improvement in mood. If you find that you're increasingly turning into a grump, you might need to spend more time in your pyjamas.

THE HEALTH COSTS

Poor sleep also takes its toll on the body. Experts now believe that getting enough high-quality sleep may be as important to your overall health as nutrition and exercise. Studies show that reducing sleep by just two or three hours per night can have dramatic health consequences. That's because sleep allows your body to restore itself and take care of vital functions including tissue repair, muscle growth and protein synthesis. Missing out on sleep can increase your chances of succumbing to a range of health problems from diabetes to death due to heart disease.[27,28] Sleep deprivation also negatively affects your immune function: one study showed that people who averaged less than seven hours of sleep a night were about three times more likely to come down with a cold.[29] The bottom line is: if you want to enjoy reasonable health, you can't afford to neglect your sleep.

SLEEP OPTIMISATION

I have a slow thyroid and can easily put on weight around my belly, but the one area in which I feel like I've won the genetic lottery is sleep. I'm one of those annoying people who is out for the count the moment their head hits the pillow. And I can sleep anywhere, too: trains, planes, automobiles, you name it. A lot of my clients are less fortunate and I know how it can interfere with their training, weight loss and general mojo. Everyone knows to avoid caffeine, alcohol and nicotine when it's close to bedtime as the chemicals in them can interfere with your sleep. If you are regularly having sleep trouble, the following basic sleep-hygiene tips might also help.

LIMIT SCREENS

How do you wind down before bed? Watching TV or mindlessly scrolling through social media are common forms of R&R before hitting the hay, but it's a good idea to try to limit your exposure to screens in the hour leading up to your bedtime. That's because the light emitted from your screen can trick your brain into thinking it's still daytime – it suppresses the production of melatonin, the hormone that regulates your sleep–wake cycles. Reading a book before you hit the light switch is a far better idea. (Particularly if it's this book.)

Most people I know use their phones as their alarm clocks, placing them on their bedside table while they sleep. The trouble is that during the night you might suddenly notice you've got a new text, email or WhatsApp message and reach for your phone, which is bad news on two counts. First, you're potentially exposing yourself to mental stimulation that could wake you up. Second, the blue light from your phone can prove troublesome.

BED IS FOR SLEEP AND SEX

The pandemic negatively impacted many areas of our lives, from our social connections to our drinking habits. Working from home also meant that for many people, the bedroom became a de facto office. Your bed may even have become a working (albeit fully reclinable) desk. That's problematic because it means that subliminally your brain might start to associate your bedroom with a place where it needs to be switched on and alert. That's not helpful when you're trying to drift off.

Make a rule to only use your bed for two things: sleep and sex. Forced to work out of your bedroom? Try using furniture to cordon off an area to delineate a separate workspace. Hopefully that'll prevent your thoughts heading towards work when they should be sliding towards sleep.

BE CONSISTENT

Your sleep is much like your training: consistency beats intensity. A lot of people white-knuckle it through the week on late nights and early starts, and then sleep late on the weekends to try to catch up. Unfortunately, that approach won't cancel your sleep debt. Research shows that our sleep doesn't like a changing schedule: study participants who cut their sleep down by five hours during the week, but made up for it on the weekend with extra sleep, still paid a cost.[30] The study showed these weekend lie-in folk consumed more calories after dinner, suffered reduced energy expenditure and experienced more weight gain. In fact, their results were just as bad as the other group who remained sleep deprived across the weekend without any catch-up sleep.

Having a regular sleep routine – i.e. going to bed and waking up at approximately the same sort of time each day – signals to your body when to wind down and perk up. The physiological upshot is that it releases melatonin at the right time, making it easier to fall asleep and stay asleep. A consistent sleep routine gives you a far better chance of getting the high-quality rest that you need.

FALL ASLEEP IN TWO MINUTES(-ISH)

If you struggle to fall asleep, try this US Navy trick that, if you practise it consistently, is meant to help you fall asleep within two minutes. The technique was popularised by famous track and field coach Lloyd 'Bud' Winter who was tasked with helping Navy pilots learn how to fall asleep quickly. Navy pilots need to have razor-sharp decision-making abilities to perform in battle, but the nature of military life meant they were often forced to adopt irregular sleeping habits. Winter's job was to try to ensure the pilots were sufficiently well-rested so they'd be on their game.

In his book *Relax and Win: Championship Performance in Whatever You Do*, he recounts that after six weeks of practice, 96 per cent of the pilots who gave this technique a go learned to fall asleep in under two minutes.[31] Here are Winter's five steps to lull your mind into oblivion:

1. Relax all the muscles in your head one by one. Breathing slowly and deeply, start by softening your eyes, then relax your jaw, and then your neck.
2. Relax and drop your shoulders, then loosen your arms and your hands and fingers, feeling the tension disappear from each muscle as you go.

3. Keep taking deep breaths, and continue on by relaxing your torso. Loosen your chest and stomach. Focus on your breath, imagining each successive breath is bringing your body to a quiet, calm state.
4. Relax your legs, from the tops of the thighs, to behind your knees, then down to your calves and your feet. Imagine your legs feeling heavier and heavier, sinking into your soft bed.
5. Finally, try to clear your mind. Imagine you're lying in a soft black hammock in a pitch-black room. Or you can visualise yourself in a canoe in the still waters of a quiet lake in the mountains. Try to let your thoughts slowly drift away. If they continue to come, repeat to yourself for ten seconds: 'Don't think. Don't think. Don't think.'

Keep practising this technique for six weeks. Even if this trick doesn't help you fall asleep in two minutes, it should help you relax and improve your efforts to drift off. It'll hopefully make you a better fighter pilot, too.

PILLAR 5

BALANCE

This part of the book was the hardest for me to write. It's the area where, sadly, I've made the biggest mistakes. Ultimately they cost me my marriage and quite a few friendships along the way. The scary thing is that at the time I was making these blunders, I was oblivious to the damage I was doing. I genuinely thought I was behaving in a responsible and conscientious way, when in hindsight I was being fatally short-sighted. I've learned from my errors and changed my ways accordingly, but my experience may still provide a cautionary tale.

Essentially, my mistake was that for many years I lost my sense of balance ... and when your balance goes, the laws of gravity declare that something is going to topple over. I put far too much emphasis on my work and my business. Investing so much of my energy there meant there was a shortfall in other life areas – namely my relationships and self-care.

What I learned through this process – and I'll get into the gory details in a moment – is that your success in life is actually made up of multiple strands. When we talk about success, most people automatically think about their professional lives in terms of work and the financial rewards and recognition it can bring. My definition of success has evolved to become much broader. My success isn't only about my work these days; it also includes my relationships, friendships and physical and mental health. Just like my business, those aspects of my life require hard work and attention if I want them to thrive (which I do!).

FOR MANY YEARS I WAS SO FOCUSED ON BUILDING MY BRAND AS A TRAINER AND DEVELOPING ACERO THAT A LOT OF MY RELATIONSHIPS SUFFERED.

Perhaps I chased professional success so hard because I'd failed to achieve my original dream of becoming a professional soccer player. Perhaps I was influenced by my parents' work ethic as first-generation immigrants. For years I lived with a rise-and-grind mindset. It got to the stage where I was working seven days a week and routinely clocking up 70-plus hours. My willingness to keep pushing and work harder than the competition even became a personal badge of honour.

I worry that our culture still glorifies that approach, too. The world has become hooked on the cult of productivity with constant exertion championed as the best way to get ahead. Think of Mark Wahlberg proudly sharing his daily schedule that involves him getting up at 2.30am, or that famous line from Dwayne Johnson (the Rock): 'Be humble, be hungry and always be the hardest worker in the room.' These are two of the most aspirational people on earth and they're not alone in promoting a lifestyle of constant hustle.

It's probably not surprising to learn that my seven-day-a-week schedule took its toll. I eventually burned out. I felt that every day had become the same; life had turned into a monotonous loop. I'd wake up (usually by 4am at the latest), train clients all day, go home, shower, eat and collapse on the couch in an exhausted heap. Then I'd repeat the process day after day, week after week.

I was so frazzled that I neglected my social life. I often felt like I didn't have the time to catch up with mates or couldn't physically muster the energy. At the time it seemed like a sensible trade-off to make. After all, I had my eyes on the prize: growing my business and becoming a success in the dog-eat-dog world of personal training. A degree of sacrifice was simply part of the deal. I built up a great gym with a client base that I'm immensely proud of. But I was so consumed with work that, in retrospect, my marriage didn't get the attention it deserved. As a result Amy and I ultimately broke up, although we remain close friends and business partners.

Looking back, I'm not even sure if my approach was best for my business, either. Don't get me wrong: a certain amount of sweat equity was obviously required to make Acero the success it is today. But when you're completely immersed in your business it can also prove counter-productive; you risk losing your broader perspective. This is something Byron Burke, a good mate of mine who also runs a business, pointed out to me. He suggested I should start to take some time off. He won me over when he said doing so would actually be a wise strategic decision. Rather than being involved in your own business 24/7, Byron explained, the smart move is often to take a step back – not only to re-energise, but to view your operation from a more detached perspective. Thinking of it in those terms I realised I could inadvertently be hurting my business, so I listened to Byron and started to change the way I went about things.

We altered the business model, focusing on team training rather than just one-to-one. I started to take Sundays off and began to feel a little better, so much so that I soon decided to take two days off a week (imagine!) as well as a couple of holidays each year. At first I was a bit nervous about stepping back in this way, but I soon discovered the business was doing better than ever – our client list kept growing and opportunities kept coming our way. That convinced me to cut my hours further and develop a more viable lifestyle. I still work hard – my first client is usually before 5am – but I also make sure I'm finished by 1pm. Then I'll go home, have lunch with my lovely girlfriend, go for a walk and have a nice dinner. I've started to rebalance my life and I'm far happier now – in part because I've made my work life more sustainable.

THE SOCIAL TRAP

Neglecting your friendships isn't just the recipe for a miserable life, it's also a dangerous approach. Catching up with your mates is a vital contributor to your overall sense of health. Studies have repeatedly shown that social connections have a major impact on your quality of life. If you haven't got friends, family or community ties, your chance of dying early may be 50 per cent higher than if you did.[32] That's why social isolation is now thought to be as bad for your health as smoking or lack of exercise.

YOUR SOCIAL LIFE INTRINSICALLY AFFECTS YOUR HEALTH, A FACT THAT CAN HARDLY BE IGNORED.

So many of us fail to get this memo and, from what I've observed, men tend to be particularly guilty. We get lazy about dedicating time and effort to maintaining friendships or trying to kindle new ones. Our social lives inevitably seem to deteriorate as we advance into our twenties and thirties. I understand how it can happen: for starters, it often becomes physically challenging as our friends become scattered further afield, move to new cities, towns or even countries due to relationships or work. Life becomes increasingly frantic at this age, too. On the work front, as you shin up the career ladder you're likely to be loaded with more responsibility, which means more time and energy needs to be expended. Parenthood can put another fatal dent in your social life. Modern dads play a more active role in their kids' lives than in previous generations, while mums are now far more likely to be combining their maternal duties with professional work. In other words, when you become a parent, especially in those nonstop early years, you're going to be at full stretch. Something has to give in the crazy juggling act between deadlines and domestic duties, and friendships are often the first to get the chop. If you've got a couple of young kids and a busy career, it becomes harder to justify catching up with mates for a surf or a schooner.

All this takes its toll. A 2019 poll in the UK found that 18 per cent of men did not have a best friend, while 32 per cent had no one they would even call a close friend.[33] The figures for women were slightly better but still alarming, with 12 per cent not having a best friend and 24 per cent lacking a close friend.

PSEUDO-FRIENDSHIPS

I believe there are certain things about the modern world that make us particularly vulnerable to isolation. Digital life makes it easier than ever for us to *think* we are getting our regular social fix, but those interactions are often a pale shadow of the real thing. Don't get me wrong – I love social media and enjoy the DMs that ping back and forth. But I'm also aware that those exchanges don't constitute a genuine social life. Digital interactions can also blind us to the fact that we're not nurturing our real-life friendships with the attention they deserve. Back in the day, you'd catch up with your mate to wish them a happy birthday. Now you kid yourself that you've ticked that box by sending them an emoji of a birthday cake. It's clearly not the same thing.

We also have pseudo-relationships with people we haven't ever met. Consider, for example, how much time you spend each month with the host of your favourite podcast. Just think about how many inconsequential details you know about them, from their weird quirks to their musical preferences. I suspect you almost certainly spend far more time with them than you do with your actual mates. That might scratch a certain social itch and give you a semblance of the camaraderie you need, but these sorts of 'relationships' only paper over the social cracks in our lives. They can never give us the same nutrient hit as genuine connection.

THE BEST THING YOU CAN DO TO NURTURE A FRIENDSHIP IS TO CATCH UP IN PERSON AS OFTEN AS YOU CAN.

If you really can't make it happen, pick up the phone to check in with a mate and have a proper conversation. I have one client who doubles down on this in a way that I love. Every weekend he'll arrange to call one of his mates, then stick in his AirPods and go for a long walk to tick off his #45daily during the chat.

LOOKING OUT FOR YOUR MATES

The worst of the pandemic may be over but I suspect many of its malign effects continue to have an impact on our lives. There's no doubt that COVID made us more insular, as we were confined to our homes and socially distanced from others. Since then restrictions have lifted and the status quo has theoretically resumed, but from chatting to clients it seems that many people haven't properly re-engaged with their broader network. Our social baseline of interaction is now lower and many of our ties feel less stable.

Our working lives have also changed dramatically. Many people now work or study from home at least some of the time. Admittedly that can be massively convenient, but it's also changed the lay of the land. After-work drinks and socialising with colleagues have suddenly become much harder. If you're only in the office twice a week you'll probably be hard at it, trying to smash through as many meetings and briefings as possible. Making the time to go for a social coffee with a co-worker is probably the last thing on your agenda. The pandemic also caused people to realign their values, meaning that many just want to get their jobs done and return to their families as soon as possible.

Another hangover from COVID is what's happened to our mental health. A 2023 University of Sydney study showed that rates of anxiety and depression have skyrocketed, with Australia now in the grips of a full-blown mental health crisis.[34] Psychologists are unable to meet the escalating demand, meaning that a lot of people are struggling with their issues alone and behind closed doors.

This unsettling backdrop means it's more important than ever for you to prioritise your social life. Catching up with a mate is good for your own mental equilibrium, and it could also be increasingly necessary for them. Most people like to put on a brave face and often it's only by chatting to someone at length that you're likely to find out if something is wrong. I'm sure your life is busy at the moment, but you can't afford not to check in with your mates and see how they're getting on. Admittedly you'll probably just wind up talking shit and having a laugh as usual, but there's a real possibility your friend might need something more. Perhaps they're facing a personal issue and need non-judgemental advice from an old mate. Perhaps they need to blow off some steam. Perhaps they're in a really bad space.

IF YOU DON'T KNOW WHAT'S REALLY GOING ON IN YOUR FRIENDS' LIVES YOU WON'T BE ABLE TO HAVE THEIR BACKS.

Everyone's life is studded with twists and turns, and if you're not there for your mates, you might well find that, when you need to count on someone, they won't be there for you, either.

HOW TO REBALANCE YOUR LIFE

Work and relationships aren't the only areas in which I've been unbalanced in the past. There've also been times when I've become too obsessive about my training. Particularly when I started in the industry, I thought the only way I could achieve the sort of lean muscularity that I wanted was by sticking to a regimen that was so restrictive the rest of my life started to deteriorate. I stopped going out with mates because I didn't want to derail my diet with beer or pizza. It'll be no revelation to learn that this path does not lead to happiness, nor is it remotely sustainable.

SO WHAT'S THE ANSWER TO THIS BALANCING ACT?

To say it's just about the binary dynamic of work-life balance is too simplistic. It's actually much more complex than that; there are multiple forces you need to consider. The best way I've heard this conundrum expressed is via the Four Burners Theory.[35] Here's how it works: visualise a stovetop with four different burners (nope, it doesn't matter if it's gas or electric). Each burner represents a key area of your life. One symbolises your work, one your family, one your social life and the final one your health. The Four Burners Theory decrees that if you want to be successful in a specific quadrant you have to turn down one of your other burners. If you want to be *really* successful in one quadrant, you have to cut off two others. Essentially, the theory is all about making trade-offs: you can't generate enough power to crank each burner to full intensity at once. Keeping two saucepans close to boiling point means the others will be lukewarm at best.

Admittedly the Four Burners Theory offers a harshly pragmatic view of life. Let's say, for example, you decide your health and your family are your two most important factors to prioritise. In that case, the theory argues, your career will take a hit and your social life will fizzle. Desperate to excel at work and clinch that fat bonus by the end of the financial year? That's all very well, but focusing on your career will inevitably cause a qualitative drop-off elsewhere.

It's a stark and unforgiving metaphor, yet I do see versions of it playing out in the real world. I've met some corporate bigwigs who've earned the huge salaries and bought the fancy properties and yachts. Financially their efforts have paid off big time, yet the sacrifices – the brutally long hours, constant phone calls and endless business trips – meant that many of them were on their third or fourth marriages. Equally, the people I know with the wildest social lives often fail to maintain the healthiest habits, meaning they don't achieve everything they want to at work, for example.

The dilemma is that each of the four burners constitutes a vital component of a life well lived.

WHEN IT COMES TO HEALTH, FAMILY, FRIENDS AND WORK, YOU CAN'T AFFORD TO IGNORE ANY OF THEM FOR LONG.

Yet the Four Burners Theory suggests that any attempt at balance means dimming your full potential elsewhere. Is there a way to regulate your energy and keep all your life saucepans nicely simmering away?

There are different approaches to this paradox. One is to accept that what ultimately stops you from pushing hard on multiple fronts is that there are only 24 hours in a single day. Time is finite but your to-do list is not. To circumnavigate this issue you can try to outsource certain responsibilities and life logistics while you devote your energies elsewhere. You might, for example, consider getting a cleaner or subscribing to a meal delivery service to free up extra time that you can then direct to one of your other burners. Working parents, for example, are often forced to 'outsource' a proportion of their domestic duties by paying for childcare to look after their kids so they can take care of their professional responsibilities.

Outsourcing can certainly help to alleviate the load but it's not a magic solution. After all, if you want to sustain meaningful relationships with your family and friends you have to put the necessary time in. It's impossible, of course, to outsource your health. If you run your own business you can recruit other people to manage some parts of the puzzle, but you still need to stay abreast of what's going on.

I've found the better strategy is a seasonal approach. It's accepting that you can't have it all at the same time. Just as nature's seasons change, so too will your life priorities inevitably grow or diminish in their importance. If you're a new parent, for example, you'll probably accept that the responsibility of looking after your baby will dominate your life for a time and that your working capacity will be diminished. If you're single-handedly trying to get a new start-up off the ground, you might accept that your weekly 18 holes of golf might be on the backburner for a while.

I've come to believe there's something in this approach, but the crucial part to remember is that seasons have to change or things ultimately go haywire. An eternal summer will lead to a nasty drought, while an endless winter is just bloody miserable. Preserving a healthy ecosystem requires the four seasons to revolve in their turn.

That's why I'm proposing a slight tweak on the seasonal approach. Personally I think you should accept that different life priorities will inevitably take centre stage at different times in your life. But you must stay mindful of what you're neglecting in the meantime so that sidelined burner doesn't completely go out. How do you do this?

I RECOMMEND CONSISTENTLY MONITORING YOUR FOUR BURNERS.

Every week, reflect on your four burners – work, health, family and friends – and mark each one with a ranking out of five in terms of your satisfaction with them. If one of those life areas happens to score under three for more than two successive weeks, you need to take action and make a concerted effort to prioritise it for the following weeks. So slammed at work that you haven't hit the gym for a fortnight? Acknowledge that reality and shuffle your priorities accordingly to free up some time to exercise. Been partying with your friends so much that so you've fallen behind at the office? Give the pub a miss this weekend and clear that backlog of work. The beauty of making these sorts of micro-adjustments is that you can keep all your burners humming along. If one burner is running low for a short time it may hardly even be perceptible to others, providing you can crank it back up and get the pan bubbling once more.

In fact, there's probably an additional lesson in here. If you can't take care of multiple things at once, when you do tackle a specific life burner make sure you attack it with all your energy. Hitting the gym? Don't mess about – go in with a plan and make that session count. Finally catching up with your best mate who you haven't seen for months? Ignore your phone for the duration of that evening and really try to connect.

It's not easy, but a successful life is about trying to pull off this complex balancing act. Maintaining the right equilibrium requires you to stay vigilant of your competing responsibilities and to regularly recalibrate your efforts. That's an ongoing challenge that you might not have even recognised in the past. Luckily, there's still time to perfect it.

IN FACT,
WHEN YOU CLOSE
THIS BOOK,
YOU CAN START.

EPILOGUE

Hopefully by this point, you're raring to go. You started reading this book with big plans and saintly intentions, and I'm hoping you still have them – just more realistically grounded.

Maybe your starting goal of losing ten kilograms in a month has smoothed out to losing a couple of kilograms; maybe it's shifted into trying to work out three times a week and make some changes in your diet, like cutting back on alcohol and getting more lean protein and wholegrains. These are all great changes; as we know by now, small and sustainable goals are more likely to succeed than big dramatic ones.

By now, you'll also have dug deep to get to the heart of what's driving you to change your life. Sometimes this can be confronting. What might have seemed like a simple desire to drop a couple of shirt sizes may be coming from deeper issues, or it may have prompted you to consider some health issues you've been ignoring. Be kind to yourself. Your body may be doing the work, but your mindset is key to staying on track.

CHALLENGE YOUR LIMITATIONS AND ONCE YOU MEET THAT LIMITATION, CELEBRATE - AND THEN PUSH THE GOAL POSTS.

Remember how I was telling you about the four-minute mile? Do you have any self-imposed limitations you're going to try to surpass? If you do (and I hope you do!), you're going to find it hard at times. Remember to take that time to prime yourself for discomfort, physical or otherwise. Get comfortable being uncomfortable, because it's often a sign of progress you should be congratulating yourself on, and make sure you have a strong routine to fall back on.

Your routine might be as simple as setting alarms to get you up earlier so you can go for a run, or it might be recording your progress every day. Be specific and realistic, and have a long-term plan, such as a 12-week workout program with clear milestones – and when you reach it, reward yourself! Keeping yourself accountable with a tracking app or posting your progress online will help keep you on track with your goals and make success feel even sweeter.

Of course, don't expect that you're not going to have some bad days, or even weeks. Life has little respect for our plans, and that's okay. Your best will always be a shifting goal post; sometimes just going for a walk will feel like a hard-earned victory.

THE MAIN THING IS THAT YOU MAKE YOUR COMEBACK BIGGER THAN YOUR SETBACK.

Dealing with these moments will be made easier if you keep yourself educated about the tools and methods you're using on the way, and try to avoid comparing your progress to someone else's, like fitness influencers who spend most hours of the day working on their strength and body, or movie stars who have professional trainers and chefs on retainer. Your progress will look different to someone else's, and though it can be frustrating, it really isn't helpful to aim for someone else's goals. And of course, be critical – the fitness industry loves to suck people in with ways and products to quickly achieve their goals.

Whether you're growing muscle, losing weight or just working on your fitness, doing your best to get 45 minutes of exercise in most days will go a long way to improving your physical and mental health. Don't forget that you don't have to be sweating buckets for your body to see the benefits – even just taking the stairs or getting off the bus a stop earlier will contribute to your overall progress.

And when it comes to your goals, don't forget to be clear about what you're trying to achieve – for example, as we know now, you can't lose fat and put on muscle simultaneously! If possible, get a professional to help figure out the best routine to meet your goals, whether it be lifting heavy and slow with fewer reps to grow muscle, or light and fast with more reps to develop power. So long as your muscles don't get bored (remember, you need to mix it up every now and then), you'll start seeing measurable results, particularly if you're employing some of that meathead mindfulness and giving your body the right fuel.

Like we saw in 'Pillar 3: Nutrition', food is a huge and wonderful part of life, and in many cases, overly restricting it can cause serious harm and long-term health issues.

TRY NOT TO FOCUS ON CALORIES SO MUCH AS FOCUSING ON SATIATING YOURSELF.

Eat mindfully, and try the *hara hachi bu* style of eating until you're about 80 per cent full. Try to keep your hydration levels up too, as we often mistake thirst for hunger. Working on hitting your macronutrient requirements will help with feeling full, and you might find intermittent fasting helps you further manage your nutrition. None of this means you can't enjoy a bit of cheeky chocolate or packet of chips, of course, but it'll help you identify when you're wanting to eat for hunger, and when you're wanting to eat for pleasure or comfort (which, if left unchecked, can become a problem).

Macronutrients aren't the only thing that will help with your goals; sleep is key, and it's easy to neglect. Whether you're a heinously early riser like me, or like a good sleep-in, the main thing is that you're getting a solid rest. It'll keep your performance sharp, help your muscles heal more quickly after a tough workout and improve your rate of weight loss – and all you have to is get a solid eight or so hours! I can't stress enough how key it is to get your Z's in.

I know this is a lot to take in – this book has likely crammed your head full of information ranging from familiar to completely foreign. Luckily, you can revisit it at anytime: there's nothing wrong with reaffirming and checking your knowledge, especially where your health is concerned. I encourage you to maybe have a chat about it with friends and family, too. A strong social network makes all the difference – rope a friend into going for a walk or workout once a week, or give them a call while you're on the treadmill.

WE KNOW NOW THAT LONELINESS IS ONE OF THE BIGGEST THREATS TO OUR HEALTH.

Besides, you might find some of your friends (especially those with full-time, sit-down jobs) might be looking to make healthy changes in their lives as well. Slogging through a workout is much easier when someone is there cracking jokes with you, after all! Not to mention, we need to keep balance in our lives; all work and exercise makes Jono a dull boy, after all.

With all this said and done, you might still be unsure where to start, or are feeling overwhelmed. There are a lot of steps, I know, especially if you're starting from scratch. Get back to those micro-goals I talked about earlier, and get some momentum going: order some gym wear; download a running app; inquire about a membership at your local gym; make some time in your calendar for a workout. These little things will add up if you keep at them.

WHAT IT COMES
DOWN TO IS THIS:
YOU DESERVE TO LIVE
THE FULLEST,
HEALTHIEST
LIFE POSSIBLE.

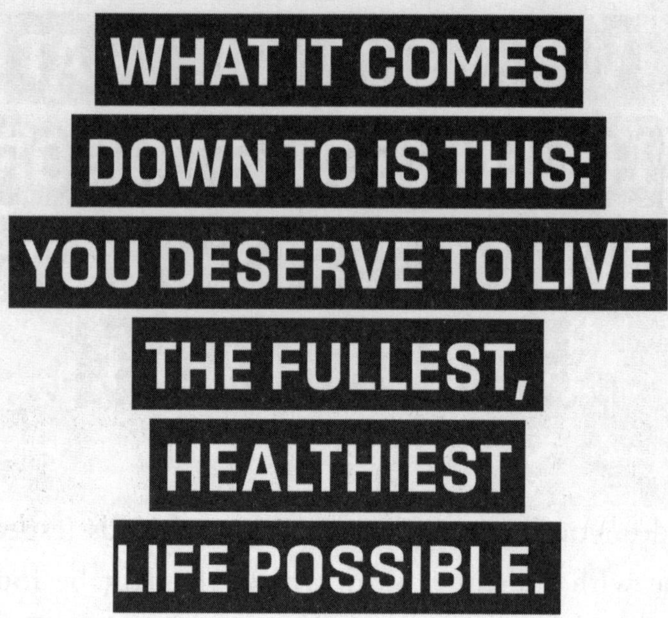

It's hard work, but it's worth it – and I think you know that, otherwise you wouldn't have picked up this book.

The next stage in your life starts today – and I'm cheering for you!

RESOURCES

WEEKLY ROUTINES

Below are two different weekly routines as an example of how strength training will differ to hypertrophy. As you can see: strength training is low rep, and would have a higher weight (I've left the weight columns blank so you can add your own); hypertrophy focuses on higher reps and lower weight. The most important thing either way is that you're using proper technique!

STRENGTH

DAY 1

EXERCISE	SETS	REPS	WEIGHT
Barbell bench press	5	5	
Dumbbell single arm shrug	4	6	
Dumbbell standing press	4	6	
Lat pulldown	4	6	
Chest press	3	6	
Elbow raises	3	6	
Wood chops	3	12	

DAY 2

EXERCISE	SETS	REPS	WEIGHT
Leg press	4	8	
Leg extension	4	8	
Goblet squat	4	10	
Single leg press	4	10	
Hanging knee raise	3	15	

DAY 3

EXERCISE	SETS	REPS	WEIGHT
Banded pull ups	5	5	
Dumbbell curls	4	6	
Seated press	4	8	
Cable knee extension	4	10	
Dumbbell elbow	4	10	
Dumbbell lateral raise	4	12	

DAY 4

EXERCISE	SETS	REPS	WEIGHT
Barbellhip thurst	4	6	
Trapbar deadlifts	4	8	
Seated leg press	4	8	
Dumbbell squat	4	8	
Hanging leg press	4	10	
Cable kick	4	15	

DAY 5

EXERCISE	SETS	REPS	WEIGHT
Barbellconventional deadlifts	4	6	
Dumbbell glute step up	4	6	
Bodyweight glute bridges	4	8	
Single arm lat pulldown	3	8	
Shoulder press	3	8	
Seated reverse fly	3	8	
Single lat raise	3	8	
T bar row	3	15	
Leg raises	3	15	

HYPERTROPHY

DAY 1

EXERCISE	SETS	REPS	WEIGHT
Barbell bench press	4	12	
Lat suprine pulldown	4	12	
Dumbbell reverse flys	4	12	
Push ups	4	15	
Single arm row	4	15	
Wood chops	3	15	
Side planks	3	15	

DAY 2

EXERCISE	SETS	REPS	WEIGHT
Barbell high bar	4	12	
Leg curl	4	12	
Leg extension	4	12	
Goblet squat	4	12	
Walking lunge	4	12	

DAY 3

EXERCISE	SETS	REPS	WEIGHT
Banded pull ups	4	12	
Dumbbell curls	4	12	
Standing press	4	12	
Seated press	4	12	
Cable knee	4	12	

DAY 4

EXERCISE	SETS	REPS	WEIGHT
Barbell hip thrust	4	12	
Bulgarian split squats	4	12	
Seated leg press	4	12	
Dumbbell squat	4	12	

DAY 5

EXERCISE	SETS	REPS	WEIGHT
Barbell deadlifts	4	12	
Push ups	4	12	
Seated row	4	12	
Dumbbell glute step ups	4	12	
Leg press high stance	3	15	
Close grip incline row	3	15	

ONE-OFF WORKOUTS

These are a collection of individual workouts you can try to spice up your routine. Use lighter weights to begin with – good technique is always key!

SHORT INTENSE
FULL BODY WORKOUT

STRENGTH

Rest 1 min 30 secs between each set

EXERCISE	SETS	REPS	WEIGHT
Barbell hip thrust	3	10	
Dumbbell Romanian deadlift	3	10	
Dumbbell chest press	3	8	
Barbell bent over row	3	8	

CARDIO

Rest 20 sec between each exercise

EXERCISE	DURATION
Dumbbell squat to press	40 SEC
Dumbbell goblet squat	40 SEC
Incline dumbbell chest press	40 SEC
Cable curl	40 SEC

[Perform 2 rounds of the above]

BACK AND
BICEPS

STRENGTH

Rest 1 min 30 secs between each set

EXERCISE	SETS	REPS	WEIGHT
Straight arm pull down	3	12	
Seated close row grip	3	10	
Pin loaded underhand lat pull down	3	10	
Seated dumbbell hammer curls	3	12	
Dumbbell hammer curls	3	12	

CARDIO

Rest 20 sec between each exercise

EXERCISE	DURATION
Mountain climbers to push ups	40 SEC
Dumbbell burpees	40 SEC
Medicine ball step up to press	40 SEC
Walkouts to push up	40 SEC

[Perform 2 rounds of the above]

BOULDER

SHOULDERS

STRENGTH

Rest 1 min 30 secs between each set

EXERCISE	SETS	REPS	WEIGHT
Dumbbell shoulder press	3	10	
Seated dumbbell shoulder fly	3	12	
Cable upright row	3	12	
Rear delt cable fly	3	12	
Single arm tricep press down	3	12	

CARDIO

Rest 20 sec between each exercise

EXERCISE	DURATION
Box jumps	40 SEC
Mountain climbers	40 SEC
Jump lunges	40 SEC
Kettlebell Russian twists	40 SEC

[Perform 2 rounds of the above]

CHEST, SHOULDERS **AND TRICEPS**

STRENGTH

Rest 1 min 30 secs between each set

EXERCISE	SETS	REPS	WEIGHT
Dumbbell chest press	3	8	
Dumbbell shoulder press	3	10	
Dumbbell shoulder fly	3	12	
Smith machine close grip bench	3	10	
Single arm tricep down	3	12	

GLUTES AND
HAMSTRINGS

STRENGTH

Rest 1 min 30 secs between each set

EXERCISE	SETS	REPS	WEIGHT
Barbell hip thrust	3	10	
Barbell Romanian dead lift	3	10	
Kettleback single rack reverse lunge	3	10	
Barbell glute bridge	3	10	
Dumbbell single leg glute bridge	3	12	

REFERENCES

1 M Rosen, 'Procrastination may harm your health. Here's what you can do', *ScienceNews*, 25 January 2023, accessed 5 June 2023. www.sciencenews.org/article/procrastination-harm-fix-resolution

2 J Scrimshire, 'EXCLUSIVE – "From what I see he is extremely happy": Matty J's personal trainer Jonathan Castano-Acero says he is "loving life" after *The Bachelor* ... as he reveals the secrets behind the star's muscular body transformation', *Daily Mail Australia*, 21 July 2017, accessed 6 June 2023. www.dailymail.co.uk/tvshowbiz/article-4716458/Matty-J-s-personal-trainer-reveals-Bachelor-body-secrets.html

3 H Chae and J Nam Choi, 'Routinization, free cognitive resources and creativity: The role of individual and contextual contingencies', *Human Relations*, 2019, 72(2):420–43.

4 M Lewis, 'You Don't Get Used to It—At Least, I Don't', *Vanity Fair*, 5 September 2012, accessed 7 June 2023. www.vanityfair.com/news/2012/09/barack-obama-michael-lewis

5 A van der Weiden et al., 'How to Form Good Habits? A Longitudinal Field Study on the Role of Self-Control in Habit Formation', *Frontiers in Psychology*, 2020, 11.

6 P Lally et al., 'How are habits formed: Modelling habit formation in the real world', *European Journal of Social Psychology*, 2010, 40(6):998–1009.

7 A Bandura and DH Schunk, 'Cultivating competence, self-efficacy, and intrinsic interest through proximal self-motivation', *Journal of Personality and Social Psychology*, 1981, 41(3): 586–98.

8 PM Gollwitzer, 'Implementation intentions: Strong effects of simple plans', *American Psychologist*, 1999, 54(7):493–503.

9 K Woolley and A Fishbach, 'For the Fun of It: Harnessing Immediate Rewards to Increase Persistence in Long-Term Goals', *Journal of Consumer Research*, 2016, 42(6):952–66.

10 C Gjestvang et al., 'What Makes Individuals Stick to Their Exercise Regime? A One-Year Follow-Up Study Among Novice Exercisers in a Fitness Club Setting', *Frontiers in Psychology*, 2021.

11 J Button, '"They cancelled me as a human": What nearly killed Logie winner Hugh Sheridan', *The Sydney Morning Herald*, 20 November 2021, accessed 7 June 2023. www.smh.com.au/national/they-cancelled-me-as-a-human-what-nearly-killed-logie-winner-hugh-sheridan-20211027-p593ls.html

12 American College of Sports Medicine, *Protein intake for optimal muscle maintenance*, 2015, accessed 7 June 2023. www.acsm.org/docs/default-source/files-for-resource-library/protein-intake-for-optimal-muscle-maintenance.pdf

13 JS Volek et al., 'Performance and muscle fiber adaptions to creatine supplementation and heavy resistance training', *Medicine & Science in Sports & Exercise*, 1999, 31(8):1147–56.

14 BJ Schoenfeld, 'Differential effects of attentional focus strategies during long-term resistance training', *European Journal of Sport Science*, 2018, 18(5):1–8.

15 RI Kingston, 'URI researcher provides further evidence that slow eating reduces food intake', The University of Rhode Island, 27 October 2011, accessed 10 June 2023. www.uri.edu/news/2011/10/uri-researcher-provides-further-evidence-that-slow-eating-reduces-food-intake

16 Harvard School of Public Health, 'Diet Review: Intermittent Fasting for Weight Loss', n.d., accessed 10 June 2023. www.hsph.harvard.edu/nutritionsource/healthy-weight/diet-reviews/intermittent-fasting

17 K Sampson, 'Late-night eating and weight gain', *The Harvard Gazette*, 4 October 2022, accessed 10 June 2023. news.harvard.edu/gazette/story/2022/10/study-looks-at-why-late-night-eating-increases-obesity-risk/
18 Australian Government, 'How much alcohol is safe to drink?', 2022, accessed 10 June 2023. www.health.gov.au/topics/alcohol/about-alcohol/how-much-alcohol-is-safe-to-drink
19 KD McManus, 'Why keep a food diary?', Harvard Health Publishing, 31 January 2019, accessed 10 June 2023. www.health.harvard.edu/blog/why-keep-a-food-diary-2019013115855
20 CD Mah et al., 'The effects of sleep extension on the athletic performance of collegiate basketball players', *Sleep*, 2011, 34(7):943–50.
21 OE Knowles et al., 'Inadequate sleep and muscle strength: Implications for resistance training', *Journal of Science and Medicine in Sport*, 2018, 21(9):959–68.
22 Kohatsu ND, et al. Sleep Duration and Body Mass Index in a Rural Population, Archives of Internal Medicine. 2006 Sep 18; 166(16): 1701.
23 *Annals of Internal Medicine*, 'Insufficient Sleep, Diet, and Obesity', 5 October 2010, accessed 11 June 2023. https://europepmc.org/article/MED/20921537
24 Csipo, T., Lipecz, A., Owens, C. et al. Sleep deprivation impairs cognitive performance, alters task-associated cerebral blood flow and decreases cortical neurovascular coupling-related hemodynamic responses. Sci Rep 11, 20994 (2021). https://pubmed.ncbi.nlm.nih.gov/34697326/
25 Harvard Health Publishing, 'Sharpen thinking skills with a better night's sleep', 1 March 2015, accessed 15 June 2023. https://www.health.harvard.edu/mind-and-mood/sharpen-thinking-skills-with-a-better-nights-sleep
26 DF Dinges et al., 'Cumulative sleepiness, mood disturbance, and psychomotor vigilance performance decrements during a week of sleep restricted to 4–5 hours per night', *Sleep*, 1997, 20(4):267–77.

27 PM Nilsson et al., 'Incidence of Diabetes in Middle-Aged Men Is Related to Sleep Disturbances', *Diabetes Care*, 2004, 27(10):2464–69
28 Lee, S., Mu, C.X., Wallace, M.L. et al. Sleep health composites are associated with the risk of heart disease across sex and race. Sci Rep 12, 2023 (2022). https://doi.org/10.1038/s41598-022-05203-0
29 MR Opp and LA Toth, 'Neural-immune interactions in the regulation of sleep', *Frontiers in Bioscience*, 2003, 8:768–79; S Cohen et al., 'Sleep Habits and Susceptibility to the Common Cold', *Archives of Internal Medicine*, 2009, 169(1):62–67.
30 CM Depner et al., '*Ad libitum* weekend recovery sleep fails to prevent metabolic dysregulation during a repeating pattern of insufficient sleep and weekend recovery sleep', 2019, *Current Biology*, 2019, 29: 957–67.
31 L Winter, *Relax and Win: Championship Performance in Whatever You Do*, Oak Tree Publications, 1981.
32 J Holt-Lunstad, TB Smith and J Bradley Layton, 'Social Relationships and Mortality Risk: A Meta-analytic Review', *PLOS Medicine*, 27 July 2010.
33 C Ibbetson, 'How many people don't have a best friend?', *YouGov*, 25 September 2019, accessed 12 June 2023. https://yougov.co.uk/topics/society/articles-reports/2019/09/25/quarter-britons-dont-have-best-friend
34 M Bower et al, 'A hidden pandemic? An umbrella review of global evidence on mental health in the time of COVID-19', *Frontiers in Psychiatry*, 2023, 14.
35 D Sedaris, 'Laugh, kookaburra', *The New Yorker*, 17 August 2009, accessed 12 June 2023. www.newyorker.com/magazine/2009/08/24/laugh-kookaburra

ACKNOWLEDGMENTS

To my beloved friends and family,

Your love, understanding and unwavering support have meant the world to me. You have stood by my side, offering words of encouragement and a shoulder to lean on during moments of doubt. Thank you for always believing in me, for celebrating both the small victories and the big milestones, and for reminding me of my potential. This book is a testament to the love and strength that surrounds me, and I am grateful beyond words.

And finally, to all my readers, followers and supporters – your enthusiasm for my work and daily posts and your kind words of encouragement have touched my heart in ways I can't express. You have joined me in this adventure, and your presence and feedback have been invaluable. Thank you for joining me on this journey, for investing your time into my story. It is because of you that my words have meaning, and I am forever grateful for your daily support. This book is dedicated to each and every one of you. You impact on my life, and I am humbled and honoured to have you in my corner daily. Thank you for being the wind beneath my wings.

With love and gratitude,

Jono Castano